PREGNANCY AND DIABETES

GW00371999

PREGNANCY AND DIABETES

Bonnie Estridge and Jo Davies

Thorsons

An Imprint of HarperCollins*Publishers*

To Suzy and Claire, for their future

Thorsons
An Imprint of HarperCollins*Publishers*
77–85 Fulham Palace Road,
Hammersmith, London W6 8JB
1160 Battery Street,
San Francisco, California 94111-1213

Published by Thorsons 1994

10 9 8 7 6 5 4 3 2 1

© Bonnie Estridge and Jo Davies 1994

Bonnie Estridge and Jo Davies assert the moral right to
be identified as the authors of this work

A catalogue record for this book
is available from the British Library

ISBN 0 7225 2959 7

Printed in Great Britain by
Mackays of Chatham, Kent

CONTENTS

ACKNOWLEDGEMENTS

The authors would like to thank the following people for their help, support and encouragement in the preparation of this book: Sue Brenchley, Kate Campbell and Dierdre Wicksley of the BDA (British Diabetic Association), Veronica Green (Diabetes Care Sister at Charing Cross Hospital), Vanessa Hilton (who typed the manuscript), Hilary Allard, Chris Butler, Chris Holland, Gloria Ferris, Dominique Giudicelli and Sarah Sutton. We would also like to thank Debbie Comber, Sandra Everton, Angela Mimms and all the other mums with diabetes who helped by contributing their experiences.

FOREWORD

In no other area of diabetes have the changes over the past decade had such a profound effect and been so far-reaching as in pregnancy. Women with diabetes can now proceed from conception to the birth of a healthy child with an optimism which was impossible ten years ago. This optimism has been brought about by the advent of accessible home blood-glucose monitoring, the use of more flexible insulin regimes and purified insulins, and the development of sophisticated scanners to monitor the growth and well-being of the baby. These developments, together with the emphasis on structured, specialised clinics and services, have been fundamental to the successes of pregnancy with diabetes.

The management of pregnancy and diabetes poses a great challenge. To be successful it is necessary to have close communication and co-operation between the woman who has diabetes, her diabetes nurse specialist, her dietician, her physician and her obstetric team. With the support and assistance of this team she can achieve the diabetes control which is so vital for the development, growth and well-being of her child.

Pregnancy for most women is a time of excitement, apprehension and joy. For the woman with diabetes, this is no different: her anxieties, however, are often far greater. She will be experiencing one of the biggest challenges of her life with diabetes, one which requires discipline and much hard work. There will be tough times, anxious times and times of frustration. But these will be paralleled with success, a healthy pregnancy and, most important of all, the birth of a healthy child.

In this book, Bonnie Estridge and Jo Davies have managed to balance all aspects of diabetes and pregnancy which are fundamental to a smooth pregnancy and the birth of a healthy child. They have done this whilst maintaining a positive and individual stance. It is written in a clear, helpful and encouraging way.

This is a wonderfully reassuring, down-to-earth, factual account of all aspects of pregnancy and diabetes and is a must for all diabetic women (and their partners) who are contemplating a family.

KATE CAMPBELL
Head of Diabetes Care and Information Services
The British Diabetic Association

INTRODUCTION

This book is about pregnancy – but pregnancy with a difference. It has been especially written for the woman who is hoping to have children or is already expecting a baby and has diabetes.

She may feel joy tinged with much apprehension and many questions as yet unanswered: Will my baby be all right? How will diabetes affect me? How can I do my best to give birth to a normal, healthy child? Can I expect a similar pregnancy to a woman who hasn't got diabetes? Can I continue my full lifestyle while I am pregnant?

The object of this book is to guide you, the mother-to-be, through pregnancy; helping you to keep healthy and stress-free while keeping your blood glucose levels under tight control. This is your key to the best chance of a good pregnancy and a healthy baby. No one can guarantee your pregnancy will be easy but the prospects are far, far better now than ever before.

There have always been risks associated with diabetes in pregnancy, but these have greatly decreased over the years as home blood-testing and a greater understanding of the condition increases. In the 1950s about 25 per cent of women with diabetes in Britain lost their babies through miscarriage or still-birth and many babies were born with birth defects. Yet today the statistics for healthy, normal babies are virtually the same as for those women who do not have diabetes – a phenomenal leap forward. Much of the credit for this is given to the realization that every effort to take tight control of blood glucose levels even before conception goes a long way towards the well-being of the baby. Perhaps a pregnancy was unplanned or you have only just discovered you are expecting a baby; right now is the time to take control and get on to the right track. Perhaps you have been told you have gestational diabetes – a form of diabetes that is peculiar to pregnancy. Although this usually disappears when the baby is born your diet will have to be reviewed and possibly changed throughout your pregnancy, with the possibility of having insulin injections if your blood glucose levels remain higher than normal.

We hope to cover everything that the mother-to-be with diabetes needs to know, from hard medical facts to diet, relaxation, help and advice for single and working mothers as well as couples. Body-care, emotional aspects, exercise, the birth and breastfeeding are also included.

Having diabetes does not mean you are an outsider to an exclusive club of perfect pregnancies (though it does mean that you will have more attention paid you than will other, 'normal' mums to be!). Each individual – with diabetes or not – and each pregnancy is unique. Everyone reacts quite differently to the experience and it goes unsaid that diabetes makes pregnancy more of a challenge. You, like everyone else, will feel the highs and lows of those long months of waiting. You may wonder how you will ever get through them. We hope that this book will help inform you and make you feel good about yourself.

Advice and understanding coupled with the benefit of others' experience will help make the most of a very personal and – one hopes – happy event.

Are you a member of the British Diabetic Association (BDA)? If not, now is the time to join – even if you have gestational diabetes and expect it to disappear once the baby is born. The BDA can provide invaluable links with others in your situation and offer support if ever you feel the need to ask advice or simply need someone to talk to. Whatever your needs from the BDA, they will ensure you never feel cut off and alone (you can find their address in the Useful Addresses chapter at the end of this book).

Chapter 1
DIABETES EXPLAINED

What Is Diabetes?

Diabetes mellitus is not a condition of modern times; it has been recognized as a serious illness for thousands of years. Attempts have been made to cure it for centuries, but it was only at the latter part of the 19th century that doctors finally came anywhere near understanding what actually caused this – as it was then – inevitably fatal condition.

Diabetes actually exists in many forms, the main two of which are:

Insulin-Dependent Diabetes Mellitus (IDDM)
Non-Insulin-Dependent Diabetes Mellitus (NIDDM).

IDDM develops in a dramatic way over quite a short period of time, whereas NIDDM has less obvious symptoms which may go unnoticed for years and are sometimes only discovered during a routine medical examination.

Diabetes mellitus results if the pancreas, a gland in the upper part of the abdomen, fails to function properly. Normally the pancreas produces insulin, the hormone which is essential for storing glucose (sugar) in the body. When a person's pancreas stops producing enough, or indeed any, insulin, diabetes

1

occurs. So instead of being burned up by the body to produce energy, the glucose remains in the blood. Without replacing insulin to process the glucose, the level of glucose in the blood rises way above the normal limit – this is known as *hyperglycemia.* [FIG1]

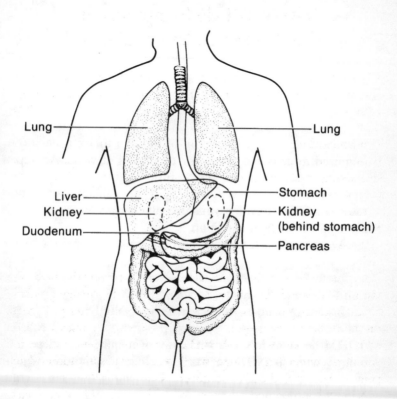

If the pancreas gland does not function properly, diabetes mellitus will be the result

The kidneys cannot cope with this overload and glucose is emptied into the urine, causing it to be sickly sweet (hence the translation of diabetes mellitus from the Greek: 'fountain of honey'). In 1679 Thomas Willis, physician to King Charles II, described the taste of diabetic urine as 'wonderfully sweet' and the condition that caused it 'the pissing evil'.

The Tell-Tale Symptoms of Insulin-Dependent Diabetes

Whether you have had diabetes for a long time or have been diagnosed recently, you may recognize some or all of these symptoms:

- burning thirst
- numerous trips to the toilet
- a strange taste in your mouth
- lack of energy
- rapid weight loss (even if you've been eating a lot)
- blurred vision
- recurrent bouts of thrush (itching genitals)

As glucose – and therefore energy – is lost from the body in the urine the body begins to 'feed from itself' by breaking down fat and protein in a desperate attempt to obtain energy. When the body fat is being broken down, poisonous chemicals called *ketones* appear in the blood. Perhaps you, or someone close to you, first noticed a strange smell on your breath rather like pear drops or nail polish remover. This is a substance called *acetone* and is due to the presence of ketones. The 'fat melt-down' – as the breakdown of fat and protein is known – also causes tiredness, weakness and irritability. If the first symptoms of diabetes (tiredness, frequent urination and unquenchable thirst) go unheeded, eventually weakness and sudden weight loss plus the build-up of ketones progress rapidly to coma and, if untreated, can lead to death (as the body has no energy left to keep going). Once treated with insulin all these symptoms quickly disappear and the patient feels miraculously restored to former health.

Before the cause of diabetes was understood, leading to the discovery of insulin, there were many weird and wonderful potions given to try and cure the disease; nothing worked. One short-term treatment was a virtual starvation diet which included boiled cabbage and water. The end result: death from malnutrition.

The first real breakthrough in understanding the condition happened during the late 1800s when doctors removed a (living) dog's pancreas and discovered that this gave the dog the symptoms of diabetes. However, they did not know exactly which ingredient found in the pancreas was missing in people with the illness. It took several decades to find the definitive connection between insulin and diabetes; in 1921 two scientists (Frederick Banting and Charles Best) working at the University of Toronto discovered the importance of insulin. It was already known that the pancreas releases essential digestive juices which enable food to be absorbed into the body. But Banting and Best's great finding was that it also produces various hormones which flow directly into the bloodstream, the most critical being insulin. By taking insulin from pigs and cows and injecting it into humans, Banting and Best found the key to treating diabetes in those who cannot produce their own insulin.

The first human to be given insulin replacement was a teenage boy who lay dying in Toronto General Hospital. Within hours of his first insulin injection he was on the way to making an outstanding recovery. Insulin replacement was seen as a miracle cure and, as those millions who owe their lives to it know, it still is.

Different Forms of Diabetes

However, as mentioned above, not everyone who has diabetes must take insulin. It is estimated that there are 750,000 people with diabetes in the UK; about one quarter of these has IDD. Once diagnosed as insulin-dependent you will remain on insulin for the rest of your life. This type of diabetes usually develops between birth and age 40, with over 3,200 cases diagnosed a year in people under the age of 20.

NIDDM is common among the elderly and those who are overweight. This form of diabetes develops because there are insufficient amounts of insulin being produced or the insulin is not working properly. Around 20 per cent of NIDDs may start treatment with dietary changes and/or tablets but later are found to need insulin injections to keep their blood glucose levels normal. Thirty per cent of NIDDMs can be treated by diet alone, and 50 per cent are treated by tablets. Gestational diabetes (described below) is often treated by diet alone, with insulin given if blood glucose levels are too high.

Tablets given to NIDDMs are not insulin, but drugs (sulphonylureas or biguanides) to stimulate the production of insulin or help the conversion of glucose into energy. Incidentally, insulin cannot be taken by mouth in tablet form as it is a protein and would be destroyed by enzymes in the stomach, hence the need for injections.

Gestational Diabetes

Pregnancy increases the need for insulin and sometimes the body cannot cope with the extra demand. Often symptoms of gestational diabetes go unnoticed as the blood glucose may be only slightly raised. Anyway, thirst, tiredness and endless trips to the toilet are part and parcel of pregnancy!

Gestational diabetes is usually picked up at the antenatal clinic after routine blood glucose and urine tests. If the blood glucose is abnormal (higher than it should be), a mini-glucose tolerance test is performed. This involves drinking a mixture of glucose and water after fasting – the mixture is warm and sickly sweet – quite revolting! Blood samples are taken before drinking the mixture and then half an hour afterwards and again another half hour after that. The samples are tested to see if too much glucose is present in the blood. If glucose levels are found to be elevated then a full glucose tolerance test (more glucose drinks and more frequent blood/urine tests) will be necessary.

Quite often pregnant women show glucose in their urine but do not have diabetes. This is because their renal threshold (that is, the level at which glucose spills over from the blood into the urine) is lowered by the pregnancy. Glucose tolerance tests establish whether a woman has an unusually low renal threshold (but does not have diabetes) or whether she has diabetes. As gestational diabetes is more likely to occur in the third trimester – the latter months – of pregnancy, high glucose levels in the early months may indicate IDDM or NIDDM in a woman who had not realized she had developed the condition.

Many hospitals are now performing routine mini-glucose tolerance tests on pregnant women at 26–28 weeks to look for gestational diabetes, but in any case the urine should be tested for glucose at every visit and, if it is found, glucose tolerance tests will automatically follow. All women who have gestational diabetes will be tested again five to six weeks after delivery to establish whether or not they still have diabetes.

The vast majority of women find their glucose levels return to normal after the birth, although a small percentage will continue to have diabetes. Gestational diabetes is likely to re-occur in subsequent pregnancies, and there is also an increased risk of developing permanent diabetes in the future for those women who have had gestational diabetes. There is nothing one can do to prevent this happening, but the risk can be lessened by avoiding becoming overweight and maintaining a healthy diet (see Chapter 6 for treatment of gestational diabetes).

Terri, aged 29, developed gestational diabetes when she was six months pregnant with her first baby. She tells us:

I had put on a tremendous amount of weight and felt very tired and thirsty. My doctor immediately put me on a diet which helped a lot as I'd been eating doughnuts every day. My weight stabilized and my blood glucose levels stayed fairly normal. I've just become pregnant again and I understand that this is likely to repeat itself, but this time I've given up the doughnuts and am trying to keep my weight within sensible limits!

Why Me?

Unless your diabetes is a side-effect of pregnancy or you were very overweight (which can stop the pancreas working efficiently) there is no real reason that can be given for what actually causes diabetes. The condition is becoming more and more common. Indeed, in the last 20 years the incidence rate of insulin-dependent diabetes in under-15s living in the UK has doubled.

In some cases it is true to say that diabetes is an inherited disorder and certain families carry a strong tendency to develop the condition (this is particularly true of NIDDM). But in many new cases of IDDM, patients are unable to trace one relative with diabetes on either side of the family. It is likely that many people carry a gene for or susceptibility to diabetes and something happens to trigger the full-blown illness. Many people believe that diabetes can develop as a result of a shock – an accident or emotional upheaval such as a bereavement – yet a shock cannot be the root cause of diabetes. Stress can only trigger a diabetes that was already developing, by changing the metabolic activity of certain hormones in the body and making the blood glucose rise.

It is possible that the cause may one day be proved to be

external or environmental. In young people it often appears to start after a viral illness or infection such as a cold, so some kind of unidentified virus may be the trigger. However, there is no such thing as an actual diabetes virus and you cannot 'catch' it from someone else. The chances of you, as a mother with diabetes, passing it on to your child are 1 in 50. If your (male) partner were the one with diabetes, the risk would be higher (1 in 20). If both of you have diabetes the combined risk would obviously be higher still. It is actually the *tendency* to diabetes which is inherited, and many children of parents with diabetes never develop the condition. At this moment in time there is no way of knowing whether, when, or what type of diabetes a child may develop. But if your child were to develop diabetes it would be extremely unlikely to happen before she was at least a year old.

There is nothing you or your parents could have done to prevent your diabetes and this will apply to you and your own children. All you can do is to try to ensure they keep a healthy diet and avoid becoming overweight (which may lead to diabetes in later life).

Modern Success of Diabetes and Pregnancy

Today, pregnancy in women with diabetes is one of modern medicine's great success stories. The survival rate for babies is almost as high as that of the general population (98 per cent). The road to a healthy baby will never be an easy, straightforward one for a woman with diabetes, yet new understanding of what previously caused such problems coupled with easy home blood-monitoring has advanced and improved matters no end.

Before insulin was invented it was virtually impossible for women with diabetes to have children. The outcome was invariably death for both mother and baby. Once insulin was

8

available the future was not quite as bleak – the mothers survived – but there was still a high infant mortality rate and at least half died. In fact, only as recently as the early 1960s, 25 per cent of these babies were stillborn or died shortly after birth.

The key to the whole problem is strict blood glucose control right from the beginning – even before the baby has been conceived. Your efforts can be helped by the many specialist centres with combined diabetes/antenatal clinics and pre-conception clinics for counselling and expert supervision (see Chapter 2).

Apart from infant mortalities it was once also the case that there was an increased risk of abnormalities in babies born to mothers with diabetes. Again, these problems have been dramatically reduced to the level found in the general population by excellent blood glucose control beginning well before the vital first weeks of pregnancy (by the end of which time the baby is completely formed).

Before we had the technology for home blood-testing, hospital tests would tell a patient very little indeed. Urine tests could be performed at home but could never give an accurate enough picture of blood glucose levels throughout the day. Mandy, who gave birth to her first child in the early 1970s, recalls:

My pregnancy was very difficult as I could never quite tell whether my glucose levels were far too high or I was about to go unconscious because they were too low. I don't remember any great importance being placed on blood glucose control except that I was told eat a lot of cheese and drink a lot of milk, presumably to fill me up so I wouldn't stuff myself full of carbohydrates.

Sarah was an extremely large baby at birth and had a few problems. She had to go into intensive care. Thankfully, she survived. I was shocked at how hazardous the whole experience had been... I never dared have another child. I'm fascinated and thrilled by how much things have changed.

9

As you will read later, better care and assessment of the baby while still in the womb are also of great benefit; hospital admissions with weeks of bed rest, routine Caesarean sections and huge, overweight babies are mostly confined to the past. The vital approach now is education of the mother-to-be, specialist care, frequent home blood-testing, eating a healthy, balanced diet and enjoying your pregnancy however hard you have to work at it!

If you are prepared to make the effort required to monitor your blood glucose levels constantly, barring unforeseen problems there is no reason why you should not carry on with your normal lifestyle. If you work and aim to carry on until your official maternity leave begins, hopefully you will be able to do just that.

As you will see in Chapter 8, sports (bar the obviously dangerous ones which are no-nos in any pregnancy) and exercise are a positive aid to pregnancy, as keeping fit helps your physical and mental welfare no end. One bold and sports-mad PE teacher – who had had diabetes for some years before the birth of her first child – tells us:

I escorted a group of schoolchildren on a skiing trip to Austria when I was four months pregnant. I deliberately left my ski-boots behind as I did not expect to ski. Loving the sport as I do, the temptation was too great and I gave in. I hired some boots and took it very gently...The fresh air, the exercise, the exhilaration...it did me the world of good...

Talk About Your Pregnancy

Never feel you should keep your diabetes a deep, dark secret. You will meet other mothers-to-be at the clinic who will be in the same boat as you and they can be valuable contacts; why not swap phone numbers or arrange to meet? Talk to expec-

tant mums who haven't diabetes as well, about *their* experiences...they will almost certainly be interested in yours. As we
said earlier, there is no such thing as a perfect pregnancy,
every woman will have her own story to tell. Sharing yours
with others can help you all.

You could also find out about local British Diabetic
Association (BDA) support groups which you might consider
joining. As a member of the BDA you will have access to
information on pregnancy, new thinking and developments;
their bi-monthly magazine *Balance* will keep you abreast of
what's going on. The BDA is unique as it is the only diabetes
organization in the world which includes patients and profes-
sionals (such as doctors and nurses) within its membership.

Diabetes and pregnancy are not ideal partners, yet with
understanding, care and self-help you can cross the hurdles
that you may feel are stretching endlessly ahead.

Chapter 2

PLANNING YOUR
PREGNANCY

Care to Expect

A baby is formed during the first 12 weeks of pregnancy (see Chapter 4). Many women do not even realize they are pregnant during these early weeks and that is why it is so very important to be prepared beforehand and ensure that your blood glucoses are controlled by the time you conceive. As some women could be pregnant for a few weeks before they have a positive pregnancy test, good control must be maintained. There can never be any guarantees that all will be perfect, but where blood glucose levels are normal at conception and then throughout a pregnancy, the risk of abnormality is a small one and, as we discussed earlier, probably the same as that for a mother who has not got diabetes.

When you have diabetes and are considering having a baby it is advisable to plan your pregnancy to give your baby the best possible chance of being healthy. The way to do this is to keep your blood glucose levels as near normal as possible before and after meals. This applies not only during pregnancy but even before you have conceived. *It is now widely recognized that good blood glucose control even before conception can minimize the risk of any problems.*

In the past women with diabetes have traditionally given

12

birth to large (*macrosomic*) babies and, though this can still happen, with good monitoring it is becoming less and less common. Macrosomia can occur if the mother's blood glucose level is too high, as glucose can pass across the placenta to the baby. If the baby receives glucose into his bloodstream, the pancreas produces more insulin to bring the glucose level down. In turn, the pancreas grows as it is then forced to produce more insulin to cope with the high glucose level; the glucose turns into fat and the baby becomes larger. A big or macrosomic baby presents a problem during labour and sometimes dies before birth. As well as being fat and 'floppy', these babies have often not developed and matured properly and therefore have difficulty breathing (in the same way that premature babies have).

Another problem these babies have is hypoglycaemia (or low blood sugar). Once the umbilical cord is cut the supply of glucose to the baby abruptly stops. However, the baby continues to produce a large amount of insulin, which then causes him to become hypoglycaemic. This can be rectified by giving the baby glucose.

Another potential complication is something called *polyhydramnios*, which is when, for some reason, the amniotic fluid that surrounds the baby (see Chapter 4) increases in volume. The sheer volume and weight of this fluid causes the amniotic sac (which contains the fluid and the baby) to rupture before the right time. This is referred to as the 'premature rupture of membranes' and can result in the baby being born premature. High blood glucose levels may also result in other foetal abnormalities such as spina bifida, heart or brain defects as well as other minor problems like an extra finger or toe.

Pre-Pregnancy Counselling

These days, many diabetes clinics run a pre-pregnancy counselling service. If you are not sure whether your clinic offers this service, speak to your diabetes specialist nurse or, if you don't attend hospital for your diabetes care, ask your GP – who will probably refer you to the hospital at this stage anyway. You will also need to attend a hospital antenatal clinic that is experienced in looking after women with diabetes. In the UK you are unlikely to find this in the private sector so it is best to attend an NHS antenatal clinic. Many hospitals have 'joint' clinics which are run by both the diabetes team and the obstetrics team. This is the ideal situation, for it means your pregnancy and your diabetes will be looked after at the same time.

I felt very apprehensive about telling my diabetes nurse that I was thinking of having a baby. I don't know why but I felt as though I wanted to embark on something that I shouldn't be doing. I didn't realize that there was any special service offered before one became pregnant and I thought there would be a lot of tut-tutting and 'do you realize what is involved,' etc. In fact, both my doctor and nurse couldn't have been more positive about the idea. They told me that my blood sugars were not quite good enough but we'd work on that. All the ins and outs were explained and I felt much more confident about everything.

You will have to give birth in hospital. This may be disappointing news if you had hoped to experience a home birth. Unfortunately, this would be too risky and both you and your baby need to be in hospital in case medical help is needed.

Although many women with diabetes are able to have a normal delivery, the need to have a Caesarean section is more likely for them than for women without diabetes. At one time women with diabetes had their labour induced early. Now women can go to full term (40 weeks), providing mother and baby are well. During labour women who have required insulin through their pregnancy will need to be attached to drips of insulin and glucose. Even if you do not take insulin for your diabetes (and are on tablets or a dietary regime alone) the baby's and your progress through labour will have to be very

14

carefully monitored. (Labour and the birth will be explained in full detail in Chapter 11.)

Getting a Grip on Blood Glucose Levels

Ideally you should try hard to gain good blood glucose control at least two to three months prior to conception, and this is where the pre-pregnancy counselling service comes in. You would normally see your diabetes specialist nurse and she would explain the importance of good control. You will be taught how to monitor your blood glucose levels if you are not already doing so. Your diabetes clinic may lend you a blood glucose meter to read your blood tests; this will give you fast, accurate results. Alternatively you could buy one (they are not available on prescription but they are now very reasonably priced). However, make sure you are taught by the nurse – and understand – how to use the meter properly, as poor technique will give you false results and mislead you. Your diet will be reviewed to make sure you are eating healthily and treatment for your diabetes will be changed if necessary (see Chapter 6, 'Treatment').

The blood glucose levels you are aiming for are between 4 and 6 mmol/l before food and no higher than 8 mmol/l one hour after food. If your control has been poor then be prepared for it to take some time to achieve these levels. But don't despair – it will be worth all the effort in the end. Your doctor and diabetes specialist nurse will also want to ensure your glycosylated haemoglobin (HbA1) is as near normal as possible before you conceive. The HbA1 is a blood test which averages out your blood glucose levels over the past two to three months. The result of this test is measured as a percentage (e.g. 6.5 per cent) and the normal range can vary from clinic to clinic. Do ask your doctor or specialist nurse the level you should aim for. At the pre-conception clinic you will also have your blood pressure checked, and the back of your eyes should be examined. Women with diabetes sometimes develop problems with their eyes (diabetic retinopathy) which can be exacerbated by the increased stress that pregnancy puts on the blood vessels. If there is any retinopathy present (extra, fragile blood vessels growing at the back of the eye) this can and should be treated to prevent leakage of these vessels. Your kidney and thyroid functions will also be assessed, along with your general state of health.

Rubella

You will also have a blood test to check your immunity to rubella (German measles). If you were not immune and were to catch this virus, especially in the first three months of the pregnancy, it could seriously damage your baby. Not only can rubella cause foetal abnormalities but also miscarriage or still-birth. If the blood test shows you are not immune then you will be vaccinated and will be strongly advised not to become pregnant for three months. If you have found out that you are pregnant but have not yet had the blood test, avoid anyone who has rubella and have a blood test as soon as possible. You may well be immune, as many girls are vaccinated routinely at school. If not, regular blood tests will show whether you have caught the virus and your doctor will discuss the implications of this with you.

You will be asked about any previous pregnancies, previous illnesses, medical or social problems you might have. If you do have any worries please don't be afraid to discuss them with the medical team. They will surely be wanting you to have a happy and successful pregnancy and are bound to do everything they can to ensure you do.

I would have liked to have known the real chances of handicap or deformity and how they were manifested. I was told there was only a slight risk of anything going wrong and no one would say anything except 'you'll be fine.' I was never given any actual statistics – which I would have appreciated – but I guess I didn't come straight out and ask.

16

Very occasionally it is suggested that a woman with diabetes should not become pregnant. This may be because she has severe kidney disease and high blood pressure or problems with her heart. Her doctor should explain the reasons why becoming pregnant would create a serious problem and give the woman concerned a chance to ask questions. Ultimately however, any decision you have to make is *your own,* and everything relevant should be discussed with your partner or those close to you and your doctor. If you are going to see the doctor for the first time it is advisable to take someone with you, as it is possible to become so engrossed in one aspect of the situation that you do not take in other details of what is being said. It is often a good idea to take notes – something you could ask your companion to do for you.

Giving Up Bad Habits

Now is the time to give up any habit that may harm your baby, once you conceive.

Smoking

There is nothing good about smoking during pregnancy. In fact there is nothing good about smoking! If you have diabetes it can cause all sorts of problems to do with your circulation and heart. If you do smoke, the following reasons should encourage you to give up:

• Nicotine can cross the placenta into the baby's blood-stream. This results in the baby receiving less oxygen and thus growing more slowly. You may think that this is an advantage, but it actually makes the baby weaker and more prone to infection. There is certainly evidence that women who smoke double the risk of having a stillborn or low birth-weight baby.

- Smokers are more likely to suffer complications such as miscarriage, bleeding or a premature birth.
- Nicotine can speed up the baby's heart rate and harm the breathing pattern of a new-born.
- After the birth a smoke-filled environment increases the risk of cot death (Sudden Infant Death Syndrome/SIDS) and the chances of your child developing ear infections and asthma.

If you do smoke, it's not going to be easy to give up. You may feel you have enough to cope with just trying to sort out your diabetes. But putting effort into your planned pregnancy should mean you go the whole way. If your partner or other family members smoke then encourage them to give up as well.

Choose a definite date to stop smoking; cutting down rarely works. Remember that exercise (see Chapter 8) helps to bring your blood glucose levels down and keep your mind off cigarettes. If you do not do any form of exercise, why not start now? It need not be anything too strenuous; walking or swimming are a good way to start.

Nicotine chewing gum or patches should *never* be used by pregnant women. And try not to munch biscuits as an alternative, this will only make you put on weight and send your blood glucose levels up. Try chewing sugar-free gum – there are many flavours to choose from and it will keep your mouth occupied! (Incidentally, sugar-free gum may also help when you feel nauseous.)

Alcohol

Heavy drinking can affect a developing baby. Indeed, some doctors believe that even a small amount of alcohol can have an effect. There is no doubt that alcohol crosses the placenta into the baby's bloodstream. Even a small amount of alcohol can impair *your* judgement, so imagine the effect this could have on a recently conceived baby! Although a small amount of alcohol only constitutes a minor risk, it would perhaps be better to give up completely.

Contraception

During the time you are trying to get your blood glucose levels under control you should use some means of contraception to prevent accidental pregnancy. Having diabetes does not mean you are any less fertile than a non-diabetic woman, but to become pregnant when your glucose levels are not controlled could lead to the problems already mentioned. There are various methods of contraception; whichever you end up with will be chosen for you as an individual and as your preference. If you are not using any contraception at the moment, your doctor will help and advise you.

Oral Contraceptives

The Combined Pill

This form of contraception combines two hormones; progesterone and oestrogen. Occasionally the combined pill can lead to changes in insulin requirements (in insulin-dependent women) but the amount would only be small. This type of pill should be avoided if you smoke (which you should not anyway!) or if you are over 35, as there can be an increased risk of the circulatory problems which can sometimes occur in diabetes. Also you should avoid the combined pill if there is a family history of heart attacks or strokes. However, side-effects have been lessened by the use of smaller doses of oestrogen in the modern pill and, if it is suitable for you, the combined pill provides an effective means of contraception.

19

The Mini Pill

This contains only progesterone and does not have the side-effects of the combined pill. Therefore it can be used by some women who have a history (or family history) of circulatory problems. The mini pill may also be used by women over the age of 35 and it does not seem to affect blood glucose control in women with diabetes. This type of oral contraceptive can also be used when you are breastfeeding. (Incidentally, it is a myth that you cannot become pregnant while still breastfeeding, you most certainly can!)

The disadvantage of the progesterone-only pill is that it is not considered to be as effective as the combined pill and should not be used if avoiding pregnancy is absolutely essential. Intermittent or 'breakthrough' bleeding may occur on the mini pill, which may cause you some worry; this should be explained to you in more detail by your doctor or nurse. However, if this type of contraceptive pill is taken on a strict, regular basis (at the same time every day, perhaps with your evening insulin if you are insulin-dependent) it can be very effective. Taking the mini pill in the evening is recommended, as it is most effective four hours after it has been taken.

It's worth remembering that there are a number of factors which may cause the pill to become ineffective. These are vomiting, diarrhoea and some drugs (antibiotics included). Do remind your doctor of any medication you may be taking and, if necessary, use barrier methods. If you forget to take your pill and are worried that you may be unprotected, family planning organizations provide specific advice on what to do, or you can talk to your GP. If in any doubt, always use a barrier method such as the sheath.

Intra-uterine Devices (IUD)

Sometimes called 'the coil', this form of contraception is mainly used in women who have already had one or more children. This is because there is an increased risk of pelvic inflammatory

disease (PID) which can lead to infertility. In women with diabetes, infection can lead to loss of blood glucose control, which
you, as a pre-pregnant woman, will be trying to maintain.
There is no proof that women with diabetes are more likely to
develop PID than non-diabetic women but bear in mind that if
any problems did occur the consequences would be more serious. This form of contraception should not be used by any
woman who has previously had PID or an ectopic pregnancy
(that is, a pregnancy formed outside the uterus – usually in the
Fallopian tubes).

Barrier Methods

Condoms (sheaths) and diaphragms (caps) are equally efficient
as methods of contraception. It is, however, advisable to use
them with a spermicidal cream. For a woman with diabetes
this type of contraception does not upset the metabolism in
any way, but it is not as effective as some of the other forms
described so there is a risk of conception at a time when blood
glucose levels are not yet under control.

Rhythm Method (Natural Family Planning)

This involves finding out when ovulation occurs and avoiding
intercourse at that time. Ovulation is the time when the ripe
egg (or *ovum*) is released from one of a woman's ovaries. This is
easier to work out if the menstrual cycle is regular, as ovulation occurs in the middle of the monthly cycle. The menstrual
cycle is usually every 28 days, although some women have a
slightly shorter or longer cycle than this. At the time of ovulation body temperature rises and there are changes in the
cervix (or neck of the uterus) that allow sperm to swim to the
egg more easily. This is the time intercourse should *not* take
place to avoid pregnancy. Some women with diabetes can
experience irregularities in their menstrual cycle which can

make the time of ovulation difficult to determine.

Contraceptive Injections

These are not often used in women wishing to become pregnant as they are fairly long-lasting. However, they can be used in women who have found other methods of contraception unsuitable or who have experienced undesirable side-effects. These injections are often used in women who have trouble remembering to take their pills. The main side-effects are irregular bleeding and an absence of periods. Temporary infertility and irregular periods may occur for a short time after treatment has been stopped, however, so even if good diabetic control has been achieved it may take a while to become pregnant and your motivation to maintain good blood glucose control could wane.

Norplant

This is the newest contraceptive device, consisting of six matchstick-sized flexible tubes placed under the skin on the inside of the upper arm (using a local anaesthetic) containing a synthetic hormone, Levonorgestrel, which is related to the natural hormone progesterone. Small amounts of the hormone are released into the bloodstream and the implants last five years. They can be removed if required and the effects are completely reversible. Norplant has little in the way of side-effects (possibly some weight gain and absence of periods) and has been hailed as 'revolutionary', 'effective' and 'hassle-free'. As progesterone is particularly suitable for women with diabetes and there is no risk of 'forgetting to take it' you may well wish to try Norplant. While it is still in its early days, one Family Planning Association report on the results of worldwide trials taken over five years found that Norplant had a failure rate of only 4 in 100, which makes it about as effective as other more established forms of contraception.

With any kind of contraception, the individual must be taken into account and there will always be a method to suit you. Your diabetes doctor or nurse or GP will discuss everything thoroughly and you should feel happy in your own mind with your chosen method.

Once your blood glucose levels are stable and your HbA1 is acceptable, your diabetes nurse or doctor will give you the go-ahead to stop using contraception. Now you can try for your baby.

How Long Will it Take to Conceive?

The length of time it actually takes to become pregnant varies enormously from woman to woman and for each pregnancy. You could conceive straight away or it may take a few months or even longer. This is quite normal.

When an egg is released from the ovary it travels down the Fallopian tube towards the womb; this is known as ovulation. The egg lives for about 24 hours following ovulation and it is during this time that it needs to be fertilized by the male's sperm in order for a pregnancy to occur. The best time to have intercourse in order to conceive is around the time of ovulation (see below). If you make love just before you ovulate, this gives the sperm a chance to travel up the Fallopian tube in time to meet the egg as it is released (sperm can survive for up to 72 hours in the womb).

By keeping a record of your monthly cycle you can work out when you are likely to ovulate. If you write down the date each time your period starts, after a few months you will be able to count the number of days between the start of your period (day one) up to and including the day before your *next* period. If your monthly cycle is regular, the number of days you have counted will be about the same. As most women ovulate about 14 days before the start of a period (whatever the length of their cycle) you can work out when you are likely to ovulate by counting back 14 days from the day your period is due. Alternatively (and some women find this easier), you can count forward 14 days from the first day of your last period. Some women experience a slight discomfort on either side of their lower abdomen when ovulation occurs.

What If Your Monthly Cycle Is Not Regular?

There are other ways to find out when you ovulate. The amount of mucus around the cervix increases just before ovulation; it also becomes thinner to allow the sperm to move through it. At this time you may notice an increase in vaginal discharge. If there is a discharge and you have not had intercourse in the previous 24 hours, it could be you are ovulating and are at your most fertile time of the month.

You can also take your temperature and fill in a chart to establish if or when you are ovulating. This method is generally used if conception is proving difficult. Your GP or family planning clinic will explain this if they feel it necessary. Sometimes, however, a woman who is not expected to conceive readily is in for a surprise:

As I have polycystic ovaries and only three or four periods a year I was given several scans and told it would take two to three years to conceive. It took four weeks!

Difficulty in Conceiving

As many women know, there is no guarantee you will become pregnant straight away. Factors such as stress, tiredness or anxiety (unrelated to either becoming pregnant or diabetes) can get in the way. If you are worried that conceiving is taking too long, do not hesitate to discuss this with your diabetes nurse or doctor. It's a sad fact of life that some women (with or without diabetes) may never be able to have children, yet there's always hope. Apparent infertility can often be resolved. A low sperm count in the man or blocked Fallopian tubes in the woman are frequently rectified. For example, if there is any indication of infertility various tests will be carried out and you will almost certainly be referred to a doctor who specializes in this field.

Missing Your Period

Once you have missed a period or even have a very slight bleed (much lighter than normal) you should have a pregnancy test. The most reliable result would be obtained about two weeks after the missed period, when a hormone called *human chorionic gonadotrophin* will have built up enough to prove you are pregnant. This hormone is the first to be produced by pregnancy and is initially responsible for maintaining it.

You will need a sample of urine passed first thing in the morning (make sure the urine is collected in a clean container). You can get your GP to organize a test for you (although it may take a while until you get the results) or go to a chemist where they perform pregnancy testing – you are often told the result within half an hour. Alternatively, ask your diabetes specialist nurse to arrange the test. You can also buy kits from the chemist to use at home, but if you do this make sure you follow the instructions *carefully* so you get a reliable result. A positive pregnancy test is reliable in 99 per cent of cases, but a negative result is not always accurate – you could still be pregnant as you may have taken the test too early. If you get a negative result from any source but do feel you are pregnant, wait for a week and do another test.

Chapter 3

NOW YOU ARE PREGNANT

Confirming Your Pregnancy

Even before you have had a positive pregnancy test you will probably experience changes in yourself which will tell you that you are, indeed, pregnant. The typical signs of pregnancy are:

- Missing a period (although there may be other reasons for this)
- Morning sickness. This is the name for the classic symptom of pregnancy, though many women feel sick from the time they wake up until the time they go to bed. Some feel sick, nauseous or actually vomit at certain times during the day. This sickness and nausea is mainly due to the high levels of the hormone human chorionic gonadotrophin which is responsible for the continuance of pregnancy. As the level of this hormone drops – by the 12th to 14th week – the above mentioned symptoms, which are often accompanied by a strange metallic or greasy taste in the mouth, usually subside. However, a very small minority of women may carry on feeling like this right up to the birth. One thing that does help alleviate discomfort for all pregnant women is frequent snacks of bland, starchy foods (see Chapter 9,

26

'How to Combat Nausea'). Obviously vomiting the food you have eaten can be dangerous and may lead to your body producing ketones. See Chapter 6 for advice on monitoring your blood glucose levels when vomiting or ill. And remember, *never* stop taking your insulin!

- Breast changes. The breasts are usually the most sensitive area at the beginning of a pregnancy. Symptoms can resemble premenstrual ones and include tingling, heaviness and tenderness. The veins may become more obvious and the nipples may stand out.
- Tiredness, sometimes overwhelming
- Passing water more often than usual, perhaps getting up during the night (although if your diabetes is not well-controlled this can also happen)
- An increased vaginal discharge which does not cause itchiness or discomfort
- A dislike for foods you once enjoyed – quite often tea or coffee

A positive pregnancy test will confirm any symptoms you may already have. Now it's up to you to maintain good blood glucose levels and give your baby the best possible start in life.

Although we think in terms of a pregnancy as lasting nine calendar months, the date of delivery is calculated as 40 weeks from the first day of your last period – that is, 280 days. Because many women do not have regular 28-day menstrual cycles, doctors call a normal pregnancy between 38 and 42 weeks, although if your doctor feels there is any risk because of your diabetes, your pregnancy may not be allowed to go more than 40 weeks.

Tell whoever has been involved in your diabetes care that you are pregnant, whether this is at a pre-pregnancy clinic or a normal diabetes clinic, and also inform your GP. Your care will now probably be taken on by the hospital but your GP may also want to be involved.

Hela attended only the hospital joint clinic for the duration of her pregnancy. Although she had 'no complaints' she does recall:

I often felt it was forgotten that I was an ordinary mum-to-be apart from one with diabetes. It would have been nice to have contact with a community midwife to ask questions which seemed too trivial to ask the doctors in the special clinic.

If from time to time you are able to attend your GP's ante-natal clinic you will indeed meet the community midwife and, if you have not met her before, your health visitor. The community midwife is trained to care for women while they are pregnant and, subsequently, their babies. You will quite often see the midwife at your GP's surgery and she will visit you at home for the first 10 days after the birth to check that you and your baby are progressing well. Then the health visitor takes over, visiting you at home and running the well-baby clinic at your GP's surgery. Both your midwife and health visitor are invaluable sources of support and information from pregnancy and the birth through to parenting a young child. This, to a pregnant woman or new mother, can be most reassuring.

If you are not in an area which runs a 'joint' clinic you will continue to see the doctor or nurse who has been advising you on your diabetes control throughout your pregnancy, even between your visits to the antenatal clinic. This is to make sure your blood glucose levels remain stable. How many times you visit the antenatal clinic will depend on your hospital, but it will be much more frequently than a woman who does not have diabetes.

Unplanned Pregnancy

But what happens if you are pregnant and the event was not planned? First of all, don't panic. Contact your diabetes doctor or specialist nurse straight away and let them know. They will see you as soon as possible and you must now start monitoring your blood glucose levels frequently. Test four times a day: before breakfast, lunch, evening meal and at bedtime; monitoring your blood glucose levels four times a day will provide a good profile of what's going on. This information is not only for the doctor or diabetes specialist nurse, but also for you.

If you are on insulin and feel confident enough, alter your doses accordingly. If you take tablets for your diabetes, continue taking them and test your blood glucose or urine frequently. Although women with diabetes who are on tablets are usually taken off them during pregnancy, you should continue to take the tablets until you see your doctor or nurse. More harm could be done to your unborn baby if you were to stop your tablets early, thus making your blood glucose level rise. Once you are taken off your tablets you will start having insulin injections and, if you do not already test your blood glucose levels, you will be taught to prick your finger and place a drop of blood on a special test strip. The results can then either be interpreted by eye against a colour-coded chart or read by a computerized meter (see Chapter 6).

After your baby is born you will almost certainly stop insulin injections and go back to the tablets. Please try not to blame yourself and feel over-anxious that because your pregnancy was unplanned your blood glucose levels may not have been as they should. Try to remember that a very high percentage of pregnancies in women with diabetes result in normal babies. Among this number are, of course, some unplanned pregnancies and women who had no pre-pregnancy counselling (although this should not be used as an excuse not to control your blood glucose levels now). The most important point, now you *know* you are pregnant, is really to try and get your blood glucose levels perfect. The sooner you do this, the greater your chances of having a healthy baby.

The Antenatal Clinic

The first antenatal clinic you will attend is the booking-in clinic. If you know how many weeks pregnant you are, this will be anywhere between the 8th and 12th week, unless you are asked to go sooner. Some clinics are infamous for their long waiting times, so take a good book or something else to keep you occupied. It's a good idea to wear clothes that are not restricting. For instance, it's a lot easier for the nurse to take your blood pressure if your sleeves are not too tight!

At this clinic and on subsequent visits you will meet:

The Hospital Midwife

As the name suggests, these midwives work in the hospital. You will see a midwife whenever you come to the hospital. Like the community midwife, hospital midwives are trained to care for pregnant women. They can deliver babies and will continue to care for you and your baby in the hospital after delivery. Hospital midwives work in the clinics, on the antenatal ward, on the labour ward and on the postnatal ward. They are experts in their field, so always speak up if you have any questions.

The Obstetrician

As you have diabetes you will always be seen by the obstetrician when you visit the clinic, to ensure your pregnancy is going according to plan. The obstetrician is a doctor who specializes in the care of pregnant women and their babies. At follow-up visits you may see familiar members of the diabetes team if you attend a joint diabetes/obstetric service.

Booking In

At the booking-in clinic you will be weighed and asked to give a urine sample. This urine will be checked for protein which can sometimes denote kidney problems, but it can also mean you have an infection which will have to be treated. At every clinic visit you may be weighed (although some clinics are phasing this out, as it does not offer a reliable guide to how the baby is progressing) and asked for a urine sample, your height may be measured and you might well be asked your shoe size (this can give an idea of whether you will be able to have a normal or vaginal delivery, as having particularly small feet can indicate that you have a small pelvic passage).

You will have your blood pressure checked, as high blood pressure could be dangerous for your baby and, from the diabetes angle, cause problems with your kidneys. If your blood pressure is regularly checked and seen to be rising then it can be treated.

Blood samples taken at the booking-in clinic and once during the third trimester will be analysed to check:

- that you are not anaemic. If you are, you may be given iron and folic acid supplements. This test may be repeated several times.
- that you are immune to rubella.
- your blood group. This is in case for any reason you need a blood transfusion. In some instances mothers may have a different blood group to their unborn baby. If the mother's blood group is Rhesus negative and the baby's is Rhesus positive, this does not present a problem in the first pregnancy. However, if a Rhesus negative mother is not given an injection of anti-Rhesus Globulin after the birth of the first baby where necessary, the second baby can become severely anaemic and very ill if the blood groups of mother and baby differ again.
- for syphilis. This is a sexually transmitted disease which has to be treated before week 20 if carried by the mother.
- for Hepatitis B. It is important to discover whether this test is positive, as special care of the baby would have to be taken after birth.
- for sickle cell disease and thalassaemia. These are diseases which can affect Afro–Caribbean and Asian people and

inhabitants of Mediterranean countries. Your baby could be seriously at risk if you have either of these conditions. If you do not know whether you are affected, do ask your doctor.

- for the herpes virus. If you or your partner have ever had herpes then you must tell your doctor or midwife. If genital herpes were to flare up during the last three weeks of your pregnancy you would probably need to have a Caesarean section, as a vaginal delivery could mean the baby becoming infected.
- for HIV/AIDS antibodies if you are in a high-risk group or request such a test.

Sometimes the doctor or midwife will also check for cancerous cells in the cervix (or neck of the womb) by performing a cervical smear. However, this is often left until after you have had your baby and then carried out at your postnatal check six to eight weeks after the birth.

The doctor will probably also perform an internal examination. This way, the size of your womb and the accuracy of your dates can be confirmed. You will be given the responsibility of looking after your own notes. After all it is *your* pregnancy and you will be expected to bring them to every appointment.

At your booking-in visit you will be asked about previous pregnancies, any illnesses (of course diabetes counts here) and other relevant information such as if twins run in your family. The doctor or midwife will ask you the date of the first day of your last period so your estimated date of delivery (EDD) can be worked out. You will also be asked questions about your occupation, whether you have a partner and, if so, his occupation. If you are a single parent you will be asked whether you live alone. The reason for all these questions is to establish whether you need help or support from the Social Services during your pregnancy. You may need to see a social worker to make sure you are receiving all the benefits you are entitled to, or to help find more suitable accommodation. If you are a single parent and live alone then it is advisable to have a contact number you can phone if you get into any difficulty with regard to either your diabetes or your pregnancy. In fact this applies to *all* pregnant women with diabetes.

Make sure you have the telephone numbers of the following to hand at all times:

- Your diabetes specialist nurse or doctor, or the diabetes ward
- A contact number on the maternity unit (ask at the booking-in clinic)
- Your GP – if there is an emergency number for calling the GP at night, make sure you have that too
- Your community midwife
- A friend or relative who is accessible and able to help you out in an emergency

If you have any worries or problems, never hesitate to ring the appropriate person. At clinic visits, always ask questions and express any worries. Making a list of notes and queries beforehand is an excellent idea and prevents you coming away having forgotten to ask half the things you'd wanted to know.

Ultrasound Scan

During your pregnancy you will have at least one or two ultrasound scans. Ultrasound gives photographic images which are formed by the echoes of high frequency sound waves bouncing off different parts of the body. Unlike X-rays, ultrasound is able to give a picture of soft tissue in detail and will print out an accurate picture of the baby in the womb.

Before any ultrasound scan you need to have a full bladder – this 'lifts up' the uterus into the abdomen and makes it much easier to see. Warm(ish!) oil or jelly is smeared over your stomach and a 'transducer' is passed over it. This small machine sends back signals which are transmitted on a black-and-white monitor screen. To the untrained eye, the picture is sometimes difficult to make out, and while the technician will probably offer a detailed explanation please do ask for one if he or she does not. This procedure is painless and does no harm to your baby. You will be thrilled to see your baby moving about, even if you cannot actually feel it at the time.

I had my first scan at 16 weeks, before I could feel any movement. It was amazing! I could see my son (although I did not know I was carrying a boy at the time). I was fascinated to see that he actually sucked his thumb.

Many hospitals will take a polaroid picture for you to take away (sometimes for a small charge) and this will certainly keep you going through those long weeks and strengthen your resolve to keep your blood glucose levels under control. (By the way, most scans cannot depict accurately the sex of your child; in any case it is the policy of most hospitals that their technicians should not 'forecast' the sex of the baby – lest they get it wrong and you demand compensation for the cost of all those frilly dresses or miniature bow-ties!)

An ultrasound scan is carried out for a number of reasons. If there is any query about dates, an ultrasound scan can give the doctor the age of the baby and the EDD can then be worked out accordingly. An ultrasound scan can also detect where the placenta is lying as well as the position of the baby. Unless there is an early problem the first scan is usually around 16 weeks (though some hospitals scan later). The scan at this time is used to check for abnormalities and is done for all women, not just those with diabetes. The type of problems that are looked for are abnormalities of the head or spine which may suggest Down's Syndrome or spina bifida. It is also possible to measure the width of the baby's neck at this time, which can give a clue to any risk of Down's Syndrome. There are also tests which provide information about the chances of your baby being a Down's Syndrome child. The second or subsequent scans may be done at any time up until delivery and are useful to check if the baby will be macrosomic or breech (lying bottom-down rather than head-down just before the birth).

Other Tests You May Be Offered

Amniocentesis

This is a test which may be offered to women over 35 (when the risk of chromosomal abnormalities increases). It can detect about 40 different abnormalities in the baby including spina bifida and Down's Syndrome. Done in conjunction with an ultrasound scan, a needle is inserted into the mother's abdominal wall and into the uterus. Fluid-containing cells discarded by the foetus are drawn off and later analysed.

Occasionally, the amniocentesis procedure can result in miscarriage; the reasons for having the test must be weighed up against whether you would be prepared to terminate the pregnancy if an abnormality was found. The sex of the baby can be detected by the cells of the skin and this may be vital if you are a carrier of any sex-linked disorders. However, doctors will never give amniocentesis simply to find out the baby's sex. The amniocentesis cannot be done until you are 16 to 18 weeks pregnant, and you then must wait three to five weeks for the results.

Alphafetoprotein (AFP)

A blood test is usually done at 16 weeks to test the level of Alphafetoprotein, a substance which is produced by the developing foetus and passes through the amniotic fluid into the mother's bloodstream. Raised levels of AFP in the blood between 10 and 18 weeks may indicate a baby with a neural tube defect such as spina bifida or some other abnormality concerning brain development. However, raised levels of AFP can also indicate a twin (or multiple) pregnancy so further tests must follow to find out what the cause actually is. A scan would probably be done to see if more than one baby is being carried and also to check your dates, as levels of AFP also rise as pregnancy progresses and a scan may show that the pregnancy is more advanced than you thought. If neither of these situations is found, a further blood test will be taken and possibly an amniocentesis. Lower than normal levels of AFP imply a risk of Down's Syndrome in which case an amniocentesis would be offered.

Chorionic Villus Sampling (CVS)

In this test a sample of the outer tissues which surround the developing embryo and placenta (the chorion) is taken by inserting a fine hollow tube and tiny syringe into the vagina and uterus. The syringe sucks out some chorionic cells and gives information on the embryo. CVS is carried out between 8 and 10 weeks to diagnose abnormalities in the embryo in women who are 35 or over or those who have a family history of genetic disorders. The results are available quickly, which is a great advantage as it gives the woman and her partner the choice of an early termination should it unfortunately prove necessary.

Incidentally, having diabetes does not provide a reason to be offered any of the above tests. The circumstances for having any of them would be no different than those for a non-diabetic woman.

Gestational Diabetes

As we discussed in Chapter 1, gestational diabetes is invariably picked up in previously non-diabetic women at the antenatal clinic during the latter months of pregnancy, usually after 25 weeks. If you have been found to have gestational diabetes then your treatment will depend on how well your blood glucose levels can be controlled by diet alone. If it is not possible to keep them within acceptable limits (the majority of women can) then you will be put on to insulin injections until after the birth (see Chapter 6).

Antenatal Classes

Most hospitals with maternity units run their own antenatal classes to help you learn breathing and relaxation techniques for the birth; this will probably be mentioned at the booking-in clinic. If going to your hospital for classes proves inconvenient, contact your community midwife who may run classes that are nearer and easier to attend. The National Childbirth Trust (a private foundation with branches all over the country) also run antenatal classes (see the list of Useful Addresses at the end of this book). You can take someone with you to many antenatal classes, so obviously the best person would be whoever is going to be beside you during the birth. This may be your partner, a relative or friend. However, if you have decided you don't want anyone with you during delivery, do not let that put you off going to a class – everyone is usually catered for! You will have to book up classes early as they are very popular. They can start from anywhere between 15 and 6 weeks before the birth.

At antenatal classes you will also be given general guidance and advice on pregnancy and labour. You may be shown a film or video of a birth and will no doubt be given a talk on breast- and bottle-feeding as well. There will also be much talk of 'birth plans' and whether or not you will opt for pain relief during labour or rely totally on your relaxation techniques. There are various methods of pain relief which may be offered to you (these are discussed in Chapter 11).

Deciding on a Birth Plan

How you would wish to give birth is to a large extent governed by your diabetes. A birth plan is your individual preference of how you would like the birth of your baby to take place. For example, you may decide you do not want any drugs for pain relief and feel you will be able to control the event by using breathing exercises. Or you may have a favourite piece of music that you want played through the delivery (although the most popular choice according to one poll is Vivaldi's 'Four Seasons', you can have pop, jazz – anything you find relaxing!)

Having diabetes means that you and your baby will be carefully monitored throughout labour. There will be wires attached to you to monitor the baby's heart and quite possibly drips of insulin and glucose into your arm. Be realistic about your birth plan: you will be restricted under these circumstances so home births, birthing pools, birthing stools and walking around the delivery room are definitely out. Please do not feel that having a 'high-tech' birth means you are missing out in any way because of your diabetes. Many non-diabetic women opt for this kind of birth and do not feel cheated by the experience.

Preparing Older Children

There is no easy way to prepare older children for the birth of a new baby. Whatever the age gap there will be some resentment however delighted your older child (or children) might seem initially. A negative reaction can be upsetting and there is little doubt that an older child will feel usurped. The best time to tell your older child is when your pregnancy is beginning to show. Nine months is a long time to a child and there really is no need to spill the beans right at the beginning, however excited you feel. When you break the news, do so honestly but gently. Remember that he or she may appear totally disinterested, especially if very young and not really able to take in the news. Make sure your other children hear the news from *you* and not by overhearing your conversation with friends. Once you have told them, talk about the forthcoming baby from time to time but, particularly if there's little or a negative reaction, don't force the issue.

Showing your other children photos or videos of themselves as babies and regaling them with amusing anecdotes of things they used to get up to will strike the right chord. Introducing them to other babies may jog their interest. A new baby will mean change: try to keep this to a minimum in your older children's lives. Make any changes you have to in advance so new routines become established before your new baby is born. For example, if your older child is going to begin nursery, ask if he can start a few weeks *before* the baby arrives. If you will not be able to take him to school and have previously done so, ask your partner (or whoever will be taking over) to introduce this change of routine sooner rather than later. Do not try to make him 'grow up' just before the new arrival is due.

> *I foolishly tried to toilet train Peter about a month before Lucy was born. I thought this would make my life easier, having only one baby in nappies. But every time I sat down to feed Lucy, Peter would want the potty, whether he needed it or not. Of course, there were times he did not ask, which made my job twice as hard.*

Make your older child feel important in helping with your diabetes. If you feel hypo (hypoglycaemic – that your blood sugars are low), let her help feed you glucose tablets or snacks. If she is old enough to recognize numbers ask her to read your blood glucose result on the meter or help compare colours on blood test strips. Playing doctor or nurse may help give a slightly resentful child a sense of importance with tasks that, as you can explain, a new baby will *not* be able to do for mummy.

As the weeks of the birth draw closer, any plans about what you intend to do with your older child while you are in hospital should be rehearsed. If she is going to stay with a relative, have some trial runs. If her father will be caring for her afterwards, a couple of days with dad (while you go out) would be a good idea. You will remain in hospital for a few days after the birth of your baby to make sure your diabetes has stabilized. Do not make any promises to your child that she can visit in case for some reason you are not up to seeing her. You may feel that seeing you and then having to leave you there in hospital will be too upsetting for her and that perhaps it will be best if she does not visit at all. However, it's usually best for a child to see mum in hospital and begin to accept the baby as soon as possible.

Buy a special present for the child to give the baby and another that you can say is especially for her from her new brother or sister. Small children may appreciate a new cuddly toy that they can feel is *their* baby. Then, when you change and feed the real thing they can be occupied with their own.

You may find *yourself* feeling more anxious than your other children are about how they will take to the new arrival! The best advice is to expect a bit of resentment and possibly some 'regressing' (it can happen that a child who was completely toilet trained or capable of dressing herself will suddenly revert to being more 'babyish' in an attempt to get as much of your attention as the new baby demands). It can help to sympathize with your other children, agreeing with them that sometimes the new baby is 'a pain' or 'always hungry' – make them your allies in coping with all the changes and you will win them over in the end.

Benefits

As a pregnant woman living in the UK you are entitled to certain rights and benefits including Maternity Allowance, free dental treatment and free prescriptions (although if you are registered as having diabetes you are granted free prescriptions for life, anyway). If you are on income support, are unemployed or on family credit you may qualify for maternity payment from the social fund and/or free glasses, milk and vitamins. Single parents may also be eligible for a tax-free weekly cash benefit (additional to Child Benefit) after the baby is born. You will find all the information on claiming rights and benefits on leaflet FB8 issued by the Department of Health and Social Security. If you are unclear exactly what you can claim for, the local Citizen's Advice Bureau or legal advice centre will help you work it out.

Working Women

So long as there are no medical reasons why you should stop work early in your pregnancy, neither being pregnant nor having diabetes should prevent you keeping your job until 11 weeks before your expected date of delivery and then returning to it 29 weeks after the birth (if you wish to do this). This is the time stipulated by law in the UK that your job must be kept open for you providing you have been with your present employer for two years full-time or five years part-time. (Please note that at the time of publication new EC laws were coming into effect that stipulated that you only have to be employed for six months full-time to be entitled to maternity leave. The Maternity Alliance (see Useful Addresses) will put you in the picture as to your individual situation.) You are also entitled to fully-paid time off to attend antenatal clinics and will be protected by law against unfair dismissal when pregnant.

Once it has been confirmed that you are pregnant, it would be wise to discuss the situation (including maternity pay) with your employer and explain that having diabetes means you will be attending antenatal clinic more frequently than would be necessary if you did not have diabetes. It is unlikely you will have any problems in this area as, hopefully, your boss will be understanding and appreciate that you are doing the best for your baby's health. You may also find that the maternity pay provided by your employer is actually more generous than the law stipulates. Some employers even offer longer maternity leave.

If you are self-employed you are eligible for Maternity

Allowance, to begin either 11 weeks or 6 weeks before your due date. This is a weekly sum payable for a maximum of 18 weeks.

Obviously if your job is dangerous in some way or unsuitable – if it involves, say, a great deal of heavy lifting or working with certain chemicals – you may have to review the situation.

It would be wise to make sure you do not have to take time off work solely because of your diabetes. Regular blood glucose checks, remembering snacks and meals and carrying glucose tablets at all times should enable you to control your diabetes at work and minimize the risk of hypos. Presumably you will be used to your routine anyway and will take it in your stride. If you are worried about any aspect of diabetes control at work now you are pregnant, then do not hesitate to talk it over with your specialist nurse.

Chapter 4

HOW YOUR BABY DEVELOPS

The First Three Months

The First Signs of Life

As we have discussed earlier, it's not uncommon to feel you are pregnant some time before your period is due. Some women claim to know days (or even hours!) after they have conceived.

I woke up in the middle of the night desperate for some ice-cream. I did a blood glucose test thinking I might be going hypo but everything was normal. I couldn't get this sensation out of my head. We had only been trying for a baby since my last period and this was it, I was pregnant.

The first weeks of your pregnancy are the most crucial stage for the baby, which develops rapidly from a fertilized egg into a tiny embryo. By the end of the third month (first trimester) this embryo will look like a tiny version of a human being.

What takes place inside the uterus throughout pregnancy is now understood as clearly as it ever will be. Yet little is known about how or why the baby develops as it does. We do know that development is controlled by the genes and chromosomes which make up the fertilized egg. These genes – half from the mother and half from the father – are the 'blueprint' or 'mas-

43

ter plan' for the physical and mental development of this new human being. But although we begin life controlled by our parents' genes, environment in the outside world (and to an extent inside the womb) can modify and sometimes completely change the effects of our inheritance. For example, a child whose entire family appears to be hopeless at any form of arithmatic can be coached to pass a maths exam at scholarship level.

During the first 12 weeks of life the embryo is particularly susceptible to outside influences and this is why poor blood glucose control, drugs, certain viruses (rubella for example) and other agents can have such adverse effects. *It cannot be over-emphasized how important avoiding unnecessary drugs and maintaining the best possible standard of health and nutrition is during the early weeks of pregnancy.*

By the beginning of the second month the egg is actually visible to the naked eye. The spine, brain, heart and other organs are forming. The head is growing faster than the body. The eyes have formed but are completely covered by the eyelids (the eyes do not open until about 24 weeks). By the end of this month the limb buds will be distinguishable and the embryo is roughly 2.5 cm/1 in long.

The Amniotic Sac

The embryo is enclosed in a bag of fluid called the amniotic sac which has developed from cells on the outside of the fertilized egg. The amniotic fluid inside the sac acts as a cushion to protect the baby if the uterus receives a blow and the baby is able to move around in the fluid, exercising her muscles and flexing her limbs. Pressure from the amniotic fluid is always towards the uterus, thus leaving the baby plenty of room to grow.

The Placenta

The placenta – or afterbirth – is the means by which the baby eats, breathes and disposes of waste products. Between them both, the baby and the placenta generate a number of very important hormones which are essential for a healthy pregnancy. The placenta grows on the outside of the membranes which surround the developing embryo, usually in the upper part of the uterus (if the placenta is found to be growing on the lower part of the uterus this is known as 'placenta previa' and requires hospitalization from 32 weeks until delivery after a definite diagnosis has been made. Painless bleeding is usually the first sign of this condition). A complicated network of vessels are formed between the mother's blood supply and that of the baby; oxygen and nutrients cross the placenta (as do certain drugs and the effects of cigarettes and alcohol).

Glucose crosses the placenta but insulin does not, which is why high blood glucose levels can affect the baby yet increasingly high doses of insulin will only affect the mother. The passage of substances between mother and baby (and their disposal) is the lifeline for the foetus. While the mother's and baby's bloodstreams are entirely separate, divided by a large number of protrusions called the villi, if the blood supply from the mother to the baby is decreased (when the mother has high blood pressure, for instance), the baby literally starves and will be smaller than it should be. A serious reduction in maternal blood flow would result in lack of oxygen and the baby could die as a result.

By the end of the first trimester the placenta is fully formed and from then on continues to grow with the baby. At term, the placenta weighs about one sixth of the baby's weight and is the size of a small dinner plate. It looks rather like a large piece of liver. When the placenta has been delivered (around half an hour after the birth of the baby) it will be examined to see how well it has functioned. Sometimes problems in the baby can be confirmed by the condition of the placenta; a small-for-dates baby may have been malnourished by a poor-quality placenta. It would be true to say that we are what our placenta made us and that each placenta is only as good as the blood supply from the mother.

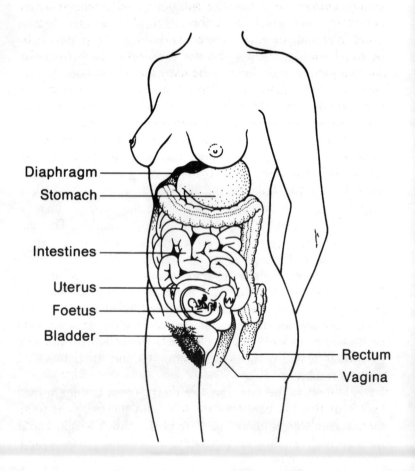

Diaphragm

Stomach

Intestines

Uterus

Foetus

Bladder

Rectum

Vagina

The foetus at 12 weeks

The Umbilical Cord

The umbilical cord is where the blood vessels in the placenta join and emerge as two arteries carrying blood to the baby and one vein carrying blood to the mother. These blood vessels are encased in a jelly-like substance and wrapped in an outer membrane which forms the umbilical cord. This stretches out from the placenta to enter the baby at the point where the navel will develop. At this site the blood vessels from the placenta join up with those of the baby and this is how the circulation between baby and placenta is completed. The baby's heart pumps blood through the umbilical arteries to the placenta and receives blood back via the umbilical vein.

The umbilical cord is about 50 cm/20 in long at term and is cut shortly after the birth. Until the cord has been cut the baby is still joined to the mother via the placenta and therefore is not a separate being or 'viable'.

From Embryo to Foetus

At 12 weeks the embryo – now called a foetus, Latin for 'young one' – is recognizably human and beginning to uncurl from its ball-like position. By the end of the 12th week the foetus measures around 11 cm/4 in and, if it reaches 13 weeks without mishap, the chances of the baby surviving to a live birth are very great. The limbs are becoming co-ordinated and strong (although you will not feel any movement just yet) and the foetus will begin to swallow some amniotic fluid, passing some urine back into the amniotic sac. Although the heart beats strongly it can, at this stage, only be detected by an ultrasound detector. The sex of the baby becomes clear as external genitals appear. Your baby will stay curled up most of the time and may suck its thumb for comfort (a habit which may still be present after the birth).

Your Blood Supply

The blood supply of a non-pregnant woman of average size has about 5 1/10 pints of circulating blood, but from about week 10 of pregnancy, this volume starts to increase gradually until it reaches a peak at around 6.5 1/13 pints and then stays the same in the third trimester. This increase in circulating blood is needed by the uterus and other vital organs. The number of red blood cells should also build up steadily, especially if a lot of iron is included in your diet.

How You May Feel

You may still be feeling nauseous or vomiting at around the 12th week of pregnancy. High levels of the hormone human chorionic gonadotrophin are in part accountable for the feelings of sickness. However, the major female hormones oestrogen and progesterone increase rapidly at this time, too. Progesterone, especially, is produced in exceptionally large quantities and is the cause of many of the initial symptoms of pregnancy, notably the enlargement of the breasts and the emotional rollercoaster you may feel you are riding at this time. Oestrogen may be partly responsible for swings in blood glucose levels in the same way as at puberty, when oestrogen levels go up and down at different times of the month, making blood glucose levels hard to control. Tiredness during this time is often overwhelming and, although your blood glucose levels will soon begin to rise relentlessly throughout pregnancy, they may actually become lower during the first trimester (see Chapter 6).

At first I had dreadful trouble controlling my blood sugars...they were up and down like a yo-yo. When I first became pregnant I found I needed more insulin (I had been told I would need less). But after a few weeks my blood sugars did drop and I had to cut my insulin dose down a lot.

The enlarging uterus starts to press on your bladder, causing you to pass urine more frequently (this is known as *micturation*) and by the end of the first trimester your clothes may start feeling a little tight.

An Emotional Experience

Of course everyone expects you to be cozily content and radiant as a mother-to-be, yet there are times when you might feel anything but! You may feel that some of the blame lies with your diabetes which could make you feel anxious about the long months ahead. However, try and comfort yourself with the thought that most expectant mums report feelings of irritability, depression and anxiety. You may find yourself inexplicably in tears despite the fact that you are thrilled to bits with yourself and your growing child. This feeling often returns a few days after the birth (and is sometimes known as 'third-day blues') when progesterone levels drop suddenly and hormone levels in the body change again. In fact, all these mood changes are largely influenced by the hormone surges going on in your body. The upheaval is so great that your feelings are, to a great extent, not under your control.

Such mood swings can last five minutes or all day, and anything can set you off. But usually that black cloud rises as quickly as it descended and everything looks rosy again.

However, although you and those around you should understand and be prepared for uncharacteristic mood swings, if you find you cannot shake off feelings of depression and gloom, don't be afraid to seek medical advice.

It's worth remembering that during the first three months of pregnancy your body is going through a major upheaval – a single fertilized cell is growing by the minute into a human being. All that has to happen after this initial period of time is that your baby has to mature, develop and grow bigger and stronger. You must look after yourself and your diabetes and let Nature do the rest. Once the first trimester is over and your hormone levels settle down you will almost certainly find that the tiredness recedes and that you feel more settled emotionally and acquire the blooming looks characteristic of a pregnant woman.

It's important to remember that in these early weeks nearly everyone has bad days (even if they won't admit it). Try not to let your diabetes make things worse by becoming depressed or exasperated at the pressures of keeping good blood glucose control; just try and focus on the end result – however far away that may seem at this stage in your pregnancy.

Try and make an effort to see others you can talk to or share your problems with. Friends with small children have been through it all themselves and can offer advice. If your diabetes specialist nurse or local BDA support group can put you in touch with a mum with diabetes who's been through it all before, you will have invaluable help. Your local National Childbirth Trust (NCT) group may even know someone who has been in a similar situation.

Rest is important, too. Take every opportunity to have naps when you can, lie-ins at the weekend (though admittedly this might be difficult if you have other children) and early nights when possible.

I was working full-time and simply collapsed when the weekends came. I had to keep setting my alarm clock for meals and snack-times or I would have slept right through them and been constantly hypo. I would wake when the alarm went off, eat and go back to sleep until the next alarm.

Remember that day-to-day anxieties will not harm your baby; although a relaxed state of mind is the ideal, it is most unlikely that the thoughts in your head can be transferred to your baby. We do know, however, that the baby in the uterus will react to physical influences from the world outside. Certainly in later pregnancy she can hear loud noises or even music in the room and even notice strong light. If you are physically agitated she may start kicking jerkily when she is stronger. Fortunately, most pregnant women become increasingly contented as time passes; their hormones see to that!

Miscarriage

It is a sad fact of life that a number of pregnancies end in miscarriage (technically known as spontaneous abortion). First pregnancies are most likely to miscarry and about one third do, sometimes before a woman even knows she is pregnant. Whether a woman has diabetes or not has no real bearing on the chance of a miscarriage, unless her blood glucose levels have been really badly controlled. Miscarriages usually happen because there is a defect in either the sperm or the ovum, thus creating an abnormality in the embryo. Sometimes the uterus has not matured enough to accept a pregnancy on the first effort. Subsequent tests on the embryo and placenta often reveal a deformity in the embryo or a placenta malfunction and it would be fair to say that this is Nature's way of preventing even further damage to the baby.

The majority of miscarriages happen during the first trimester when the baby is actually developing (after the 28th week the death of the foetus is known as a stillbirth). The first signs of miscarriage are vaginal bleeding, often with stomach cramps and not unlike a heavy period. Sometimes in early pregnancy slight 'spotting' of blood may occur and although this usually stops soon after it began it is wise to lie down and take things easy. There is no real way of knowing whether a miscarriage is going to happen; the best advice must be to call your doctor and go to bed. If you pass any clots, membranes or even the foetus and placenta, they must be collected in a clean container as they will need to be examined. Do not take any medication until you have seen the doctor and then only act on his or her recommendations.

If a miscarriage is 'threatened' – there is bleeding but losing the baby is not inevitable – you will be advised to have complete bedrest until the bleeding has totally subsided. Once the blood supply to the uterus has increased you will be able to get up but you should take extra care not to exert yourself until you have felt the baby move (at around 20 weeks, if this is your first baby). There are many different types of miscarriage and the emotional effects can be devastating.

I lost my third baby at 10 weeks. I was taken into hospital and after the miscarriage I was on a kind of 'high' for some days. It's hard to explain but I felt as though I'd actually given birth to a live baby. I was told that this was due to sudden hormonal activity. I came down to earth with a bang when all those extra hormones had disappeared and felt terribly low for weeks. I blamed my diabetes, of course, yet all the medical team assured me that examinations carried out showed that this was almost certainly not the case and I had been well controlled. I felt like giving up but within two months I was pregnant again and now I have the daughter I longed for. This second pregnancy was strong, with no threats of history repeating itself.

Always take medical advice for treatment following a miscarriage and, unless you are advised otherwise, believe it when you are told that there's no reason you should not try for another baby. Unless there are medical reasons why you should wait, sexual relations can resume when the bleeding has stopped. It is perfectly normal to feel anger, grief and depression...perhaps even guilt, however groundless. Try to talk about your feelings and, however much you may want to be alone and brood, don't confine your emotions to yourself. Counselling is extremely helpful at such a time – don't be afraid to seek help.

Chapter 5

YOUR GROWING BABY

The Rest of Pregnancy

The Second Trimester

The middle three months of pregnancy are usually those in which you feel the most comfortable, energetic and relaxed. Hormone levels will have settled down now and, hopefully, you will feel healthy and vigorous.

By **13 weeks** your baby is completely formed; now it will steadily grow and mature. By **week 14** there will be a distinct increase in the weight of the foetus. The head of the foetus is still large in proportion to its overall size (around 10.5 cm/5 in), but the body is rapidly catching up. All major muscles now respond to motivation from the brain. Elbows bend, fingers curl and make fists.

By the beginning of the fourth month the movements from the baby are vigorous as its muscles get stronger and stronger. If this is your first pregnancy it is unlikely that you will actually feel the baby kick at this time, though subsequent babies are usually felt after about **16 weeks**. The body of the foetus is now covered with a fine, downy hair called *lanugo*, and the eyebrows and eyelashes start to grow. You will almost certainly look pregnant now, with a fast-disappearing waistline.

By **week 20** you will probably have felt foetal movements. These can feel almost like air bubbles popping or butterflies.

Some women even liken them to a 'windy' feeling! It's a good idea to note the date you first felt your baby move in case there is any question about over your delivery date. Now that the baby is growing so rapidly – length about 25 cm/10 in – you will notice that the bulge caused by the enlarging uterus rises to the level of your navel or just above it and your weight will increase steadily. Your baby's teeth are forming in the jawbone and hair is growing on his head.

Insulin requirements usually start to increase around this time, although some women's fall again before delivery. The placenta produces hormones which have the opposite effect to insulin on glucose levels and it is thought that an increase in these hormones is the reason that extra insulin can be needed. Yet a small number of women do not need any more insulin during pregnancy and their placental hormones are found to be quite normal. Apart from this theory (which has not been conclusively proven) researchers still do not fully understand why insulin requirements should change during pregnancy.

During the middle of my pregnancy I needed about 100 units of insulin by day and 20 at night as opposed to my normal dose of 20 by day and 12 at night. Multiple injections with a pen certainly helped. I was offered an insulin pump but I resisted this, as being a PE teacher it would not have been practical to have a permanent needle attached. [See Chapter 6 for more about insulin pumps.]

By **week 24**, the end of the second trimester, you may feel your baby hiccuping; you may also be aware if he coughs. By the end of this time your baby will measure about 33 cm/13 in. The area around your nipples (the areolas) will be more prominent, changing from pink to brown in colour. Some women start producing colostrum (or 'milk') at this time. By now your heart and lungs are working overtime, some 50 per cent harder than normal. Increased blood circulation may make you feel flushed and hot, and your face may become puffy if you are retaining fluid.

Although the baby now has all the organs that he needs to

survive in the outside world they are not sufficiently developed to function properly if he were to be born now. There is also little fat under the skin and he would not be insulated enough to keep warm. The chances of survival if born at this stage are poor as the baby would be too premature to survive even in an incubator...however, with modern technology a number of babies have survived, albeit against the odds.

The Third Trimester

By the **28th week**, the baby's head is more in proportion to his body and fat stores are now beginning to accumulate. He measures about 37 cm/15 in in length and is now filling a lot of space in the uterus. Whereas before he was swimming and kicking freely in the amniotic fluid of the womb he will soon be finding it difficult to turn around. The body is covered in a thick soapy substance (the *vernix*) which prevents the skin from becoming clogged up with amniotic fluid. The skin is wrinkled and red and the baby's head and limbs can easily be felt through the mother's abdominal wall at this time; an ordinary foetal stethoscope can now be used to hear his heart. The lungs are now reaching maturity and, by the end of the 28th week, the baby is deemed legally viable (that is, capable of living independently of the mother, if given special care).

You may notice that your baby's behaviour is forming a pattern. He will almost certainly have periods of activity followed by quiet, though it is not known whether babies actually sleep in the womb. As the uterus grows, the skin on your stomach will begin to stretch and feel tight. Your breasts may have started to produce colostrum (the first milk, which is a light yellowy colour – see Chapter 12). Do not squeeze the breasts, simply wipe any leakages away with a tissue.

By **week 32**, the baby's proportions are much the same as they will be at birth and he is much stronger. His movements are vigorous and, in most cases, his head will be pointing down towards the pelvis. The uterus rises to meet the rib cage and your 'bump' will be getting larger and larger. As your internal organs come under pressure from the growing uterus you may feel the need to urinate frequently or may suffer from indigestion.

The placenta has now reached maturity and if born now the baby would have a 50 per cent chance of survival. His length is roughly 40.5 cm/16 in. You may start feeling more sluggish as the ensuing month progresses and your ankles may swell at the end of the day due to fluid retention. By the end of the eighth month the baby's skin has changed from a reddish colour to a more recognizable shade, as fat begins to be laid down under his skin, and his digestive system is maturing.

At or around **week 36** the baby's head – if it is pointing downwards – descends into the pelvis (if this is your second or subsequent baby this occurs much later and often not until labour has actually started). This is known as 'engaging'. Once the head is engaged you will notice that your 'bump' drops and the pressure is removed from the ribcage, making you less prone to heartburn and indigestion. Do not worry if the baby's head has not descended at this stage, there is no cause for concern; even some first babies don't engage right up until the onset of labour.

During the next month the baby will gain 28 g/1 oz a day and will fill the womb with no room to manoeuvre. You will a notice a definite difference in his movements – they will feel more like prodding or digging than flutters. Sometimes you can see the definite outline of a foot or an elbow as it nudges the wall of the uterus and protrudes beneath the surface of your stomach. Many babies' eyes are blue (but may change colour a few weeks after birth); the nails are soft and feel like skin.

You may also notice your uterus hardening with what are known as practice – or Braxton Hicks – contractions in readiness for delivery. Braxton Hicks contractions are a normal phenomenon of pregnancy which occur about every 20 minutes throughout the nine months. However, they become stronger and more noticeable towards the end of term so are often mistaken for the real thing. Their function is to aid the foetus by squeezing out stale blood from the uterus walls which then refill with fresh blood. If you do become confused as to which are the contractions of true labour, remember that Braxton Hicks are not usually painful (though you may feel a slight discomfort), are shorter in duration and not as frequent as the real thing. Braxton Hicks contractions are useful for practising breathing techniques.

During the last month the uterus rises again (having dropped when the baby's head engaged) as the baby puts on a final growth spurt. The baby is now fully developed and his length will be around 51 cm/20.5 in. His organs are able to function and all his reflexes are working. He can see, hear and smell and his voice is ready to make itself heard as soon as he takes his first gulp of air. The amount of greasy vernix will have decreased and there will only be some residue left in the folds of his skin. The baby's movements may be uncomfortable for you now as he squirms, barely able to change position in the womb.

The baby at 40 weeks

All is now ready for labour to start and even though the estimated date of delivery you will have been given is 40 weeks after the start of your last period, it is unusual for babies to arrive on time. Some are early, some are late – though as you have diabetes it is possible that your doctor will prefer you not to go beyond term. To err on the side of safety, he or she may want your labour to be induced (see Chapter 11). Your baby's movements will probably continue up until the start of labour; a sign of imminent birth is often a noticeably less vigorous baby.

I was encouraged to keep my blood sugars even lower than normal during the last couple of months of my pregnancy. This, I was told, was to prevent any risk – however slight – of the baby becoming too large at the last moment, so to speak. I have to say, I got incredibly fed up of my frequent hypos, trips to the toilet and my baby daughter lurching in my stomach at all hours of the day or night. Then, all went quiet. Suddenly I was in hospital and a few hours later there she was. Every hypo, kick and blood test was absolutely worth it!

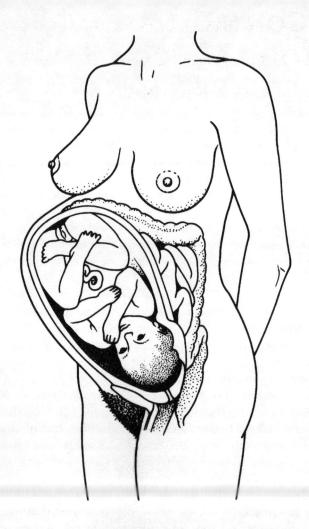

The baby at 40 weeks

Chapter 6

CONTROLLING YOUR BLOOD GLUCOSE LEVELS IN PREGNANCY

Treatment

Keeping your blood glucose levels tightly controlled is absolutely vital in pregnancy. This will be achieved either by intensive insulin therapy (altering insulin frequently to cope with rising glucose levels) or really strict attention to your diet. If you have gestational diabetes you are more likely to be treated by dietary methods alone, but if controlling your diabetes proves impossible with dietary changes alone then it's likely you will be started on insulin injections until the birth. Once your baby has been delivered, your blood glucose levels should return to normal and insulin can be stopped.

For most women gestational diabetes is only a condition of pregnancy (that's why it's called 'gestational'), yet there are some who do go on to develop true diabetes. For this reason, if you have had gestational diabetes you will be given a glucose tolerance test (see Chapter 1) five to six weeks after you have had your baby. This will show whether or not you actually still have diabetes.

During pregnancy, insulin requirements increase considerably and a woman with diabetes who is taking insulin at the beginning of her pregnancy may find that by the time the baby is ready to be delivered the amount of insulin she is taking has doubled or even tripled. If you find your insulin requirements increasing dramatically, don't worry: the actual amount of insulin required is irrelevant as there is no set dose; it's a very individual issue. So long as your blood glucose levels are controlled it does not matter how many units you are taking.

I had been used to around 50 units a day, but by the time my son was born I was on 250. I lived at the pharmacy, waiting for prescriptions.

It's amazing that the minute the baby is delivered and the umbilical cord is cut, insulin requirements go back to normal. In the case of gestational diabetes this usually means insulin is no longer needed. Women who usually take tablets for their diabetes can go back to taking their original medication (unless they are breastfeeding, as the effect of the tablets can pass through breastmilk and cause hypoglycaemia in the baby; in this case insulin treatment may have to carry on until the baby is weaned).

Different Kinds of Insulin

There are many different types of insulin which work in a variety of ways. They fall into specific categories: clear, cloudy, and bi-phasic (a mixture of clear and cloudy) insulin.

Clear Insulin

This type of insulin is also referred to generically as soluble, regular, short- or quick-acting. It looks like water. Clear insulin begins to work half an hour after it has been injected and is most effective between two and four hours after injection. After that its effect diminishes until it has been absorbed, after between eight and 10 hours. As blood glucose levels are highest after food, clear insulin is the type that works on a meal (such as breakfast) soon after it has been injected. If you are on multiple injections, clear insulin *only* will be injected before meals, cloudy insulin before bed.

Cloudy Insulin

This is opaque and looks much thicker than clear insulin. Cloudy insulin falls into two sub-categories:

1. Intermediate or medium-acting (isophane). Once injected this starts to work after about one to two hours and can work for up to 24 hours. Its peak is between six and eight hours after injection. Therefore, when injected before breakfast it begins to work mid-morning and peaks at the same time as the rise in blood glucose after lunch. It then continues to work as a background insulin, covering the afternoon snack and working until the evening meal, before which another injection may be given. Medium-acting and short-acting insulin can be mixed together if required; the way these insulins work will coincide with the rise and fall in blood glucose levels throughout the day.
2. Long-acting insulin. This is also cloudy but works for up to 36 hours. Again, it is usually used in combination with clear insulin.

Bi-phasic Insulin

This is a ready-made mixture of clear and cloudy insulin; it is also known as a fixed mixture. This type of insulin is cloudy in appearance and comes in different ratios of clear to cloudy such as 10/90, 20/80, 30/70, 40/60 and 50/50. The amount of short-acting, clear insulin is always written first on the bottle.

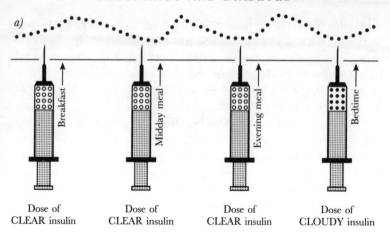

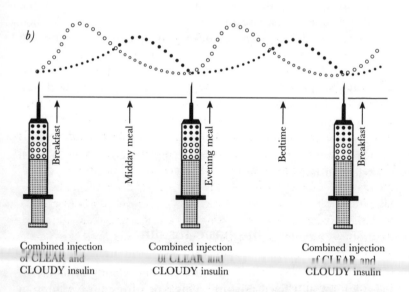

a) Small doses of clear, short-acting insulin peak just after mealtimes; a dose of cloudy insulin before bedtime will last through the night. b) Bi-phasic (mixed clear and cloudy) insulin ensures peak as well as background levels of insulin.

Insulin is measured in units and you inject what the doctor or diabetes specialist nurse suggests, adjusting the dose if necessary to control your glucose levels to within the range advised by your clinic. By frequent home blood-testing you will be able to monitor your control and, on the basis of results, make decisions on altering the dose to get things right.

If you have had diabetes for some time and are already taking insulin, you will no doubt know how to increase or decrease your insulin dose according to your blood glucose levels. However, always contact your clinic if in any doubt whatsoever. If this is all new to you, don't worry. Be led by your doctor or specialist nurse and, if there is ever anything you don't understand – please ask. You'll be surprised at how soon you become your own expert and take things completely in your stride.

How Many Injections?

The number of injections you happen to have has no bearing on how 'good' or 'bad' your diabetes is – there is no such thing as good or bad diabetes, but there *is* good and bad control. As you are trying to achieve good control, the number of injections it takes to get this is the right number for you. Many clinics prefer pregnant women to inject four times a day. This means injecting short-acting insulin before each meal (breakfast, lunch and dinner) and a medium-acting insulin before bed to last overnight. You may think that injecting four times a day sounds a daunting prospect but this actually makes it easier to alter any particular dose to control blood glucose levels throughout the day. Some clinics are happy to let you inject two or three times a day; it all comes down to how well you are able to control your blood sugars.

When to Inject

Insulin should be injected 15–30 minutes before breakfast and before your evening meal if you are having two injections a day. Four-times-a-day insulin should be given 15–30 minutes before each meal and then once before bed. If the time between having the insulin and eating the food is greater than 30 minutes, blood glucose levels could fall too low before the food has been absorbed and lead to a hypo during or after the meal. If the time between taking the insulin and eating is too short then the food could be absorbed and raise blood glucose levels before the insulin has had a chance to act. Of course, sometimes it's just not possible to leave the right gap before food, especially if you are not eating at home. For instance, if you went out for a meal, ordered your food and injected, problems could arise if the service was slow and the order took ages to arrive. So, if you are not at home it is safer to inject as you see your meal arriving. (Incidentally, if your meal does take a long time to arrive and you have already injected you can always ask for some bread or orange juice to keep you going.) If you should forget to take your insulin altogether until you are halfway through your meal or even afterwards, don't panic, just take it as soon as you remember.

Ways of Giving Insulin

Syringes are made from disposable plastic; the BDA suggests that each syringe can be used for up to five injections. After this the needle may become blunt and so cause pain when you inject. There is no need to clean the needle after use as there can be no risk of infection, but be sure to replace the cap. Syringes come in three sizes: 30, 50 and 100 units. Each line on the 100-unit syringe represents two units while each line on the 50- and 30-unit syringes represents one unit, so always check which kind of syringe you are using.

When you are first put onto insulin injections you will be taught how to draw up insulin correctly either from a single bottle or from a mixture of the insulins in two bottles.

'Pens'

'Pens' are injection devices that, as the name suggests, look just like a cartridge ink or fountain pen. They are made of hardened plastic and look completely inconspicuous. You unscrew the pen and simply fit in a cartridge of insulin which, depending on how much insulin you need, generally lasts a few days. The 'nib' of the pen is the needle, which you change after every few injections. At the top end of the pen there is a dial which clicks as each unit of insulin is measured. The more units of insulin you dial, the more the button at the top rises. There is a little window in the pen so you can see how much you have dialled. When you reach the correct dose, press the button and the insulin is delivered.

One word of warning – at the time of writing pen needles are not available on prescription in the UK (unlike the syringes), so if you choose to use a pen device you may have to pay for your own needles (the pen itself is available free from the hospital or your GP). The BDA are fighting to get pen needles on prescription as they are so widely used.

There are also disposable pens available which hold considerably more insulin than the cartridge type and contain the insulin in a pre-sealed cartridge within the pen unit. The needles can be changed as necessary; once the insulin is used up you throw the whole device away.

Insulin Infusion Pumps

Insulin infusion pumps are another way of delivering insulin directly into the body throughout the day, when required. A pump is a small device worn outside the body, either on a belt or a shoulder-holster. Inside the pump is the insulin, which is expelled through a fine plastic tube. The tube is attached to the body (usually at the stomach) by a small needle through which the insulin passes. The pump provides a continuous flow of insulin which the wearer can control. This is particularly useful at mealtimes – the wearer has only to press a button to allow more insulin to pass down the tube to cover the rise in blood glucose which will occur following the meal. However, these pumps are no longer manufactured in Britain (although existing ones can be repaired if necessary). A few women we spoke to were put onto pumps by their diabetes clinics for much of pregnancy and managed to achieve good control.

I needed so much insulin that I would have had to have continual injections. The pump sorted out the problem although I have to say it was extremely irritating and there were many times when I felt like ripping it off. I'd go through it again, though – I had a healthy, beautiful baby boy.

Injecting for the First Time

If being pregnant means this is the first time you will be giving yourself insulin by injection, you may well be dreading it. Yet the thought is invariably worse than the deed. There are some people who really do have an injection phobia and if you suffer from this you will probably be given help by a psychologist if your doctor thinks it necessary. In fact the majority of people do manage to cope well, especially if they know they will only have to have injections for a short while. You do not inject into a vein, just into the fatty tissue under the skin. The needle is short and designed not to go in too deeply. Make sure that you do not always inject into the same place. If you always use, say, one small area on your leg, the skin may become hard and lumpy and the insulin will not be absorbed at the correct rate.

Insulin is absorbed at different rates depending on where it is injected. It is absorbed most rapidly from the abdomen, then the arms, then the thighs and buttocks. You may not like the idea of injecting your stomach with a baby inside – but it is perfectly safe as the short needle could not possibly do any damage. Vigorous exercise and heat speeds up the absorption, so don't inject before a bath or shower thinking you will have your meal afterwards, as the heat from the water will make your veins dilate. Your insulin will start working faster than you anticipated and could cause a hypo.

Insulin injection sites

If you are about to do your first injection, try to find somewhere quiet where you can be alone, and *take your time* – there's no need to hurry. You don't need to clean the skin with any swabs or spirit as this only toughens it up making it more difficult and painful to inject.

Choose your site, then, holding the syringe between your thumb and forefinger, use your other hand either to stretch the skin at the injection site (if there is enough there) or gently pinch the skin between your thumb and forefinger to form a mound.

Push the needle in all the way to the hilt. If you don't push the needle in far enough then a lump may form under the skin (if this does happen, don't worry – just remember to push the needle in further next time).

If you notice a little insulin has leaked out of the injection site, do not try to make up for the loss by giving yourself more – you have no idea how much has leaked out and it would only be a tiny amount in any case. Just stop any further leakage by pulling the skin to one side, thus sealing up the injection site. Leakages sometimes happen, so please don't worry. If you accidentally hit a small blood vessel you may notice a spot of bleeding – this may cause some slight bruising but is harmless and nothing to worry about.

When using a pen injector, simply dial your correct dose, use the same technique to push the needle in your skin and press the button down smartly. Incidentally you *can* inject through clothes, but this will blunt the needle more quickly.

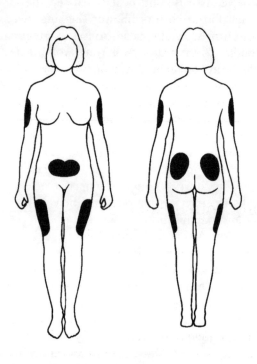

Insulin injection sites

Human Insulin

'Human insulin' is synthetic (man-made) from bacteria and is chemically identical to insulin found in the human pancreas. It is made under sterile conditions and cannot cause any infectious diseases. Before Human insulin was produced, insulin was obtained from the pancreas of pigs and cows. Although this insulin was similar to that of human beings it was not as good a match as synthetic insulin.

There have been reports that a small number of people noticed a change in their hypo symptoms when they switched from animal to Human insulin. If you are just starting insulin therapy you will be started on Human insulin so this problem will not arise. Human insulin is preferred in pregnancy as it has less antibodies than animal insulin. You will learn to recognize your own hypo symptoms from the start. If you have been changed from animal to Human insulin and are not happy about it, do speak to your doctor. Animal insulin is still manufactured so you could change back. The insulin used for pen devices is Human insulin only; animal insulin is not available for the cartridges.

Adjusting your Insulin to Control Blood Glucose Levels

Blood tests at home are vital. You can only tell just how much insulin you need by testing your blood glucose levels frequently. Now you are pregnant, the more tests the better to keep tight control. The hospital or clinic will tell you how often to test and what the levels should be. The sort of levels you should be aiming for are between 4 mmol/l and 6 mmol/l before meals and no higher than 8 mmol/l 1 hour after meals. You will probably be advised to test before each meal and before bed every day. Testing after meals sometimes will give you a good idea of how well the dose is covering the meal. If you have previously tested your urine you will be told to switch to blood tests during your pregnancy, as urine tests cannot possibly give an accurate enough picture.

The big advantage of testing your blood is that it shows exactly what your blood glucose level is at the precise time you test. The information is completely up to the minute, unlike urine tests which give 'old news'; urine in the bladder is likely to have been there for a couple of hours, so if your blood glucose level was high at any point within the past few hours then glucose will have spilled over into the urine. Also, you may have a low renal threshold (see Chapter 1). Having instant information at your fingertips (literally!) can only help you; once you have been testing for a few days you will know how much insulin you need – then, if ever you have a high or low result you can adjust the level accordingly.

Testing your blood glucose levels

If you have never tested your own blood before, your diabetes nurse will show you how to do it. You just prick your finger using a small needle or 'lancet' especially designed for this purpose. The easiest way of doing this is with an automatic device which looks like a pen and pricks the skin with speed and minimum discomfort.

By pricking the skin (the tough skin around the sides of the fingernail is best – as with injection sites you may want to change the finger you use often to avoid hardening of the skin and loss of sensitivity) you obtain a large enough drop of blood to cover a test pad (found on the blood testing strip). There are several brands of these strips available and you must follow the instructions carefully on whichever type you choose. You will get your result within 12 seconds to two minutes depending on the brand and whether or not you use a computerized meter which measures the blood glucose electronically. This cuts out the need for timing, wiping the strip or having to compare the result to a colour chart. There are several electronic meters on the market but these are not available on prescription in the UK (though the test strips are) and have to be bought. Your diabetes nurse may show you various models that you can try out before deciding which one to buy. If possible, buy a meter; they speed things up considerably. Some models have recently become very reasonable in price. If you cannot afford one, ask your diabetes specialist nurse if she has one you could borrow during your pregnancy.

Your insulin requirements will rise as your pregnancy progresses – particularly in the second half (see Chapter 5) so it is very important to keep up frequent blood tests right the way through until delivery, thus giving your baby the best possible chance of being healthy.

Long-term Blood Tests

When you attend the clinic your doctor will talk to you about one of two blood tests, either a glycosylated haemoglobin (HbA1) or a Fructosamine. These tests show your average blood glucose levels over the past two to three months (HbA1) or two to three weeks (Fructosamine). These tests even out the peaks and troughs of your blood glucose levels and give a broader picture. However, even though you have these tests this does not mean you can forget about home tests. The day-to-day picture is just as important and by adjusting your insulin to give good results on a regular basis you can ensure that the long-term picture is a good one. When you conceived, your HbA1 should have been in the normal range (every hospital has its own 'normal range', so ask for yours) and this normal range is what you and the medical staff will be aiming for right the way through pregnancy.

When You Are Ill

You must *never* stop taking your insulin – whatever the circumstances. That includes times when you are ill, even if you are vomiting and cannot eat. Illness can cause a rise in blood glucose levels and you may actually require *more* insulin, not less. If you really feel too ill to eat, take your carbohydrates to

TESTED BLOOD GLUCOSE LEVELS
(in mmol/litre)

MONTH		TEST TIME						
Day	Date	Before B/Fast	After B/Fast	Before Lunch	After Lunch	Before Dinner	Evening	Before Bed
Mon	1	4·2	7·6	5·2		5·6		9·5
Tues	2	3·8		4·5		4·8	✷4	8·6
Weds	3	2·2	1·7	8·2		6·5		7·0
Thurs	4	5·1		4·8	8·1	6·6		8·1
Fri	5	4·5		6·0		(9·2)		6·3
Sat	6	5·2		5·8		(11·1)		5·6
Sun	7	4·4		3·2		8·1		7·2
Mon	8	5·6		6·2		4·8		6·3
Tues	9	6·1		3·8		5·8		4·8
Weds	10	4·1	8·2	6·2		4·8		(3·4)
Thurs	11	5·2		6·0	7·9	6·2		(2·8)
Fri	12	4·5		5·5		4·5		9·5
	13							
	14							
	15							
	16							
	17							
	18							
	19							
	20							
	21							
	22							
	23							
	24							
	25							
	26							
	27							
	28							
	29							
	30							
	31							

BLOOD GLUCOSE MMOL/l

20-
15-
10-
5-
2-
0-

INSULIN
DOSE GIVEN

INSULIN		COMMENTS
AM	PM	REACTIONS, MEDICATION, ILLNESS, ETC
6/6	8/15	
		Hypo before breakfast ＊
6/8	8/15	Increased lunch time dose as previous days pre-dinner too high
6/8	6/13	Figures too low before bed – couldn't eat enough dinner so decreased pre-dinner insulin
DIET:		＊ Had to drink milk and glucose so level after breakfast high ＊＊ Forgot bedtime snack – explains hypo next morning KEEP OFF CREAM CAKES!

balance your insulin in liquid form such as fruit juices, non-diet fizzy drinks, Lucozade or milk. Test your blood glucose levels every two hours and increase your insulin if you have to. You should also test your urine for ketones using the appropriate strips, which you use by dipping in a sample (or your stream) of urine. Compare the colour pad on the strip to the chart on the bottle and, if you are showing any ketones at all, contact your diabetes doctor or nurse immediately. As we explained in Chapter 1, the build-up of ketones in the blood can be very dangerous and can cause weight loss, vomiting and drowsiness resulting in coma if the correct action is not taken. Ketoacidosis can also be fatal to the foetus.

You *must* contact your diabetes doctor or nurse if you are ill and:

- cannot control your diabetes
- show ketones in your urine
- are vomiting.

Do not hesitate to act if you are at all worried, as prompt action could prevent a crisis.

You need to maintain your carbohydrate intake if you are ill. If you cannot face proper meals, here are some suggestions to keep you going. Each of the following contains 10 g of carbohydrate:

Lucozade	50 ml/2 fl oz
Fizzy drink (non-diet)	100 ml/4 fl oz
Milk	200 ml/7 fl oz
Fruit juice	100 ml/4 fl oz
Non-diet yoghurt (half a pot)	50 g/2 oz
Ice cream	50 g/1 oz
1 pear, orange, apple	
1 small banana	
Sugar or glucose	2 level teaspoons/ 2 lumps
Glucose tablets	3 tablets

Some people notice a rise in blood glucose levels even if they just have a cold, whereas some have little or not trouble with illness. Again, everyone is different and all women have different reactions and needs. This also applies to hypos, which will be discussed in the next chapter.

Chapter 7

HYPOGLYCAEMIC EPISODES ('HYPOS')

How Likely Are You to Have Hypos During Pregnancy?

As any person with insulin-dependent diabetes (and some tablet-takers) will testify, hypoglycaemia or insulin reaction is an 'occupational hazard' which they strive to avoid. The most common causes of hypoglycaemic episodes or 'hypos' are:

- missed/late meals or snacks
- injecting too much insulin
- exercising without reducing insulin or taking extra carbohydrate.

Balancing food, insulin and exercise is the key to keeping glucose levels within a normal range, yet sometimes levels fall for no apparent reason during pregnancy. If early warning signals (such as feeling dizzy, sweating or trembling) are ignored or missed then glucose levels will continue to fall and a severe hypo may occur, leading to total confusion and bizarre behaviour. At worst, the hypo-sufferer may lose consciousness and even fit.

Initial hypo warnings are very individual; most people recognize their personal symptoms immediately yet some are not aware until the hypo has advanced and find themselves unable to act in time (though this is fairly unusual).

Kathy's personal warning sign is a tingling around the lips:

I feel as though I've got pins and needles...I keep wanting to rub my lips together. As soon as I feel this coming on I eat something sweet. If I do a blood sugar test, sure enough it's pretty low, usually around 2.5 mmol/l.

All people with diabetes who take insulin or certain diabetes tablets may have mild insulin reactions and feel the need to eat something sweet to raise a low blood glucose level at some time or another. A severe reaction (that is, one which necessitates help from another person to inject glucagon – see page 83 – administering glucose gel or getting you to hospital) is a more uncommon occurrence.

The same applies in pregnancy: the majority of pregnant women who have diabetes have little or no problem with hypos. However, overall, there does seem to be a higher frequency of severe hypos in pregnancy than for people with diabetes who are not also pregnant. A small number of pregnant women appear to be prone to repeated episodes of hypoglycaemia – one doctor reported a personal record-holder who had used 60 glucagons during one pregnancy! However, cases like this are very much the exception and, although it seems that hypos during pregnancy occur more in women who had many hypos before becoming pregnant, it is still almost impossible to predict who will have this problem and there are exceptions to every rule and generalization.

When Hypos Are More Likely

Forewarned is forearmed, so it's worth noting the phases of pregnancy during which hypos are most likely to occur.

In very early pregnancy, from a few days after conception

until around 16 weeks your insulin requirements may drop considerably because of low blood glucose levels. After this period, the placenta produces hormones which have the opposite effect to insulin and it is quite normal to need increasingly higher doses of insulin (thus making hypos more unlikely). In the last few weeks of pregnancy hypos may occur (more commonly at night) and may carry on to delivery, during labour and sometimes immediately after delivery.

During the last weeks I had a pattern of 1 a.m. hypos which usually woke me up and could be resolved by frenzied chocolate eating! Once or twice I actually became unconscious and my husband had to bring me round with Hypostop *[a thick glucose gel available from chemists and on prescription]. We could never work out why this was happening...I had made sure my sugar levels were good at bedtime and that I had eaten a long-lasting starchy snack and even reduced my evening insulin. It just didn't seem to add up. I wondered whether the baby (who kicked incessantly all night) was using up my energy supplies! My doctor said that perhaps this was the case, but admitted that no one really knows the reason.*

A very small number of women are unfortunate enough to suffer hypos throughout their pregnancy, but these are certainly in the minority.

Why severe hypos should occur during pregnancy is not understood. The only obvious factor would be the tight control of blood glucose levels that pregnant women are urged to keep. If you are aiming at an average of 4.5 mmol/l there are bound to be times when your blood glucose levels drop too low. In early pregnancy the inability to eat a required amount because of nausea or actual vomiting may mean your carbohydrate intake is not matching the amount of insulin you are injecting and this could cause hypos. If this is the case, try to make up your carbohydrates with drinks such as fruit juice or milk.

Hormones may play a part in causing sudden swings in blood glucose, as the levels of so many different hormones change during pregnancy. However, which hormones – if indeed any – cause unpredictable swings and why some women are affected and not others remains a complete mystery. There have been findings which point towards the fact that in late pregnancy some women become ultra-sensitive to even low levels of insulin during the night but not during the day (which could explain the more common occurrence of night-time hypos). But at this point we are no further in understanding why these changes in insulin sensitivity should come about at all. The only circumstance of which there is some understanding is labour, where energy is expended because of contractions of the womb and thus blood glucose levels (and therefore insulin requirements) do drop. After delivery, once the placenta is removed insulin requirements fall very sharply as the hormones produced by the placenta, which have the opposite effect to insulin, are no longer there. Very occasionally a mother with diabetes does not need any insulin at all for some days after delivery, which is another of life's little mysteries.

I had been up to almost 150 units of insulin a day before Jonathan was born. Suddenly the nurses told me there was no need for injections and I thought 'this is it, having a baby is the cure for diabetes...' But of course, within two days I was back on my pre-pregnancy dose (around 50 units). Of course I was disappointed but too excited by my new baby to really care that much.

Watch for Warning Signs

Sometimes personal warning signs change during pregnancy; again, doctors have no explanation for this. At worse, hypos can strike suddenly and with no warning at all; this, naturally, can be frightening.

However, serious consequences to the mother from hypos

are very rare (drinking alcohol and becoming hypo could well be an exception to this, as alcohol lowers the blood glucose and may block the release of glucagon from the liver – another good reason not to drink!) The best you can do is monitor your blood glucose levels closely at the recommended times (see Chapter 6) and even more frequently if this brings you a feeling of security. If blood glucose levels are averaging around 2 mmol/l then reduce insulin until your blood glucose levels are around 4 mmol/l. Make sure you eat and drink enough carbohydrate to balance the insulin (if you are worried that you are not eating enough, speak to your diabetes specialist nurse or dietitian). If you find yourself going hypo at night try different bedtime snacks or lowering your insulin.

I seemed to wake feeling hypo at 2 a.m. every night. In the end I pre-empted this by setting the alarm for 1.30 a.m. and having a little feast of toast and marmite...That sorted things out!

Making sure you eat meals and snacks at the right time will help considerably. The majority of hypos occur because timing of food intake has been left too late to coincide with insulin peaks.

You can also make hypos less of a problem by:

- Making sure everyone who knows you and spends time with you understands what diabetes means and how to identify and treat a hypo if necessary. Always wear ID, preferably in the form of something that is always on you, such as jewellery.
- Making sure you never sleep through a meal or snack time. You are bound to be tired and want to sleep, but set an alarm to ensure that you do not skip a meal.
- Asking a partner, relative or friend to 'check up on you' at times of the day or night when you might be alone. If you live alone, perhaps you could arrange for a relative or friend to make contact with you at a certain time every morning. You may feel this is unnecessary fussing and that

you have coped well with your diabetes until now, but this is a time when you are particularly vulnerable so don't be too proud or stubborn to ask for some help.

- Never driving before a meal or snacktime. If you have no problems with hypos and check your blood glucose levels before setting out on every journey there is no reason why you can't continue driving a car. However, never take to the road before a mealtime, carry glucose both in the car and in your pocket or bag, and never drive for more than two hours without a snack. If you feel early warning signs stop immediately, move into the passenger seat (so the police cannot book you for driving without due care and attention – that is, while hypo) and have some glucose...don't continue your journey until you have done a blood test to ensure everything is back to normal. Carrying spare blood-testing equipment in the car would be a good idea in case you forget to take your everyday equipment out with you. If you are suffering from hypos it would certainly be wise to give up driving while you are pregnant.

- Trying not to worry or get stressed out about something that may never happen. The majority of pregnant women with diabetes do not suffer from bad hypos and you may worry yourself sick for nothing. Take every precaution possible but think positive and try to relax.

Hypos and Your Baby

Please do not worry that hypos – even frequent and/or severe ones – will harm your unborn baby. Mothers who have experienced hypos during pregnancy give birth to normal babies who suffer no ill effects. Sometimes in late pregnancy hypos may cause the baby's heart rate to slow down but this recovers as soon as the hypo in the mother is treated – and no problem to the baby results.

In actual fact, the majority of mothers who have problems with hypos during pregnancy seem undaunted by history repeating itself and inevitably go on to have subsequent children. It may be comforting to learn that one extremely eminent doctor in the field of diabetic pregnancy, Jorgen Pedersen of Sweden, has made his findings known that, in his wide experience, expectant mothers who have hypos in early pregnancy (while the baby is at the formative stage) are the least likely to have abnormal babies, probably because hypos are an indication that the mother's glucose levels are near normal. It has been found again and again in research around the world that the higher the mother's HbA1 the more likelihood of abnormalities in the baby. So, it is surely worth keeping blood glucose levels under tight control, braving the thought of hypos (while doing everything within reason to avoid them) and knowing that you are doing your very best for your baby.

Treating Hypos

If you feel early warning signs, treat an impending hypo immediately with glucose tablets, a sweet drink or your favourite chocolate (though chocolate may not be absorbed as rapidly as liquid or tablets). A general guide is:

- 10 g of quick-acting carbohydrate, e.g. 50 ml Lucozade,
- 100 ml non-diet fizzy drink,
- 2 level teaspoons sugar, honey, jam or syrup, or
- 3 – 4 glucose tablets.

Follow this up with 10 g of a longer-acting starchy carbohydrate to keep glucose levels up (otherwise they may fall again):

- one slice of bread,
- a digestive biscuit, or
- a small bowl of cereal.

Your relatives, friends and workmates should know that a severe hypo should (ideally) be treated orally with a sweet drink such as Lucozade (always keep a small bottle handy at home or in your desk at work). If you cannot take liquid – and it is very dangerous to give liquid to someone who is unconscious – whoever is with you should be able to lay hands on *Hypostop*. This thick glucose gel is sold in a plastic bottle with a spout. You squirt the Hypostop into the side of the mouth and rub the cheek (it is absorbed through the cheek lining). Hypostop is available from most chemists and the majority of doctors in Britain will prescribe it on the NHS.

If there is no way of bringing you round orally, *glucagon* will have to be used. Glucagon is a hormone which works in the opposite way to insulin. When injected into the body it stimulates the liver to release its own supply of glucose. Although you may never need it, you should have an up-to-date injection kit handy should your hypo be impossible to treat in any other way.

A kit of quick-acting glucagon comprises two small glass bottles – one with powder, the other with sterile water. It also contains a plastic syringe. Draw up the water using the syringe, then inject the water into the bottle containing the powder. Shake the bottle to allow the powder to dissolve, then draw up the mixture back into the syringe and inject under the skin in the same place and using the same technique as for injecting insulin.

Obviously you will not be doing this yourself so it's important that your partner or whoever is with you the most knows what to do should the need arise. It's worth getting an out-of-date kit from your GP or hospital and letting your partner (or whoever) have a 'practice run' so he or she knows exactly what to do. You should put instructions on the glucagon kit that, in the event of your not coming round in 10 to 20 minutes after glucagon has been given, the doctor or ambulance should be called as it may be necessary to give glucose directly into a vein.

Do not worry if you are sick after being given glucagon, this is a common occurrence. A few people have even reported being sick after taking Hypostop. However, make sure you eat some starchy carbohydrate once you come round to maintain the glucose level, as the effect of quick-acting glucose does not last very long and levels could fall again thus causing another hypo. Incidentally, being a naturally acting hormone (like insulin) glucagon causes no harm to mother or baby.

The information in this chapter has not been written to worry you or cause you to panic. As mentioned before, it's the minority who have any real problem with hypos while they are pregnant. But for those who may be unlucky enough to suffer from them, it's important to know that there *are* ways to cope.

Chapter 8
KEEPING FIT AND RELAXED

Exercise and Sport

Unless your doctor has told you otherwise (if there has been a threatened miscarriage, for instance) there is no reason why you should not exercise during pregnancy. Pregnancy and labour call for stamina and make great demands on the body so you need to be in good shape both physically and mentally. Depending on the sport or activity – providing it is neither too vigorous nor in any way dangerous – it can be carried on throughout most of your pregnancy as long as everything is progressing normally and your doctor agrees to it.

Exercise is positively beneficial for keeping blood glucose levels under control (so diabetes is no excuse for inactivity!). Indeed, providing you take precautions to stop your blood glucose levels dropping too low (drop your insulin dose or take extra snacks before working out) you will be doing yourself a real favour by making every effort to stay fit. A sensible rule is to follow your habits rather than to change them, so barring the obvious you will be able to continue many activities that you enjoyed before you were pregnant even if the pace has to become more sedate. However, if you have done little or no exercise previously, now is hardly the time to take up squash, tennis or step aerobics. You can, however, start toning yourself up gently: walking, swimming or exercises especially designed for pregnancy will make you feel more lively, less lumpy and make it easier for you to get back in trim after having the baby.

Some forms of exercise (such as yoga) do not require energy as such, but do remember to check your blood glucose levels before and after anything you do that requires exertion. Depending on the effort required, take 10–20 g extra carbohydrate or give yourself less insulin – and bear in mind that some types of exercise may lower your blood glucose for up to half a day afterwards so you may need extra snacks to compensate.

Also remember...

- Rest comes before exercise during pregnancy – if you feel tired, take it very easy.
- If any exercise feels uncomfortable, or makes you feel nauseous, dizzy or in any pain, STOP. Don't resume activities until you feel completely well again.
- Washing floors, vacuuming and making beds are vigorous duties in themselves so don't over-tire yourself with housework and then rush off to a keep-fit class.
- The heart has to work harder during pregnancy and actually enlarges with the increased load, so don't give it unnecessary work by going beyond your capabilities.
- Always keep glucose tablets handy in case you feel hypo.
- If you already attend or are about to join a class, make sure the instructor knows you are pregnant and have diabetes, and always carry ID (preferably in the form of a necklace or bracelet) stating you have the condition.

Going to Classes

There are many types of antenatal exercise classes which you can join. Some are organized by the local hospital or clinic, some are run by private associations such as the National

Childbirth Trust (NCT), and many leisure centres, health clubs and individual teachers offer exercise classes designed especially for pregnant women. If you have been going to classes and prefer to continue with these you should take their suitability into account. High-impact aerobics, vigorous bending and stretching or step classes would cause too much strain, although if you are particularly experienced and fond of a certain class it may be possible to modify certain exercise sequences and leave out sections that could cause problems. Take advice from your instructor as well as your doctor as soon as you know you are pregnant. Low-impact aerobics, traditional keep-fit and non-acrobatic dance classes should be fine, but always consult your doctor first.

Relaxation classes such as yoga are ideal, although even simple-looking poses can put quite a strain on the body if you are a novice. Again, check with your doctor.

Exercise and Relaxation Programme

You can do all the programmes outlined below in your own home. They are designed for pregnancy but, especially if you have never exercised before, you should always begin with breathing exercises. Remember whenever you get up off the floor to roll onto your side first. Feel free to do these gentle exercises to the music of your choice.

Relaxation and Breathing

Hand Press
Apart from being relaxing, this exercise is good for your stomach muscles, breasts and upper arms.
- Stand straight with your hands together in a prayer position in front of your chest, shoulders dropped and elbows lifted outwards.

- Breathe in (slightly slower than normal breathing), expanding your stomach muscles.
- Then breathe out, pulling your stomach muscles in (as much as is possible!) and pressing the palms of your hands together as hard as you can.
Repeat 10 to 20 times.

Deep Breathing

Deep breathing is a very good way to relax; this exercise is also good for your tummy.

- Lie on your back on the floor in a relaxed position, with your knees bent upwards and feet slightly apart and with your hands resting on your stomach.
- Breathe in slowly, making the breath as long as you can manage and expanding the stomach: feel it rise with your fingers.
- Then, breathe out slowly, emptying your lungs, pulling your stomach flat (again, as flat as possible!) and pressing the small of your back into the floor. Start by breathing out to a count of 5 and work up to 10.
- Repeat the exercise 10 to 20 times.

Stretch

This is both a relaxing and stretching exercise.

- Sit on the floor with your legs stretched out in front of you, knees together and back straight but relaxed.
- Breathe in, lowering your chin forward so that you lengthen your spine (but keep it straight), at the same time reaching upwards with your arms – the palms facing each other and fingers splayed.
- Keeping your legs straight and your arms in the same position, stretch out forward from the base of the spine, simultaneously breathing out and pulling in your stomach.
- Lean as far as you can over your legs and hold it for a few seconds before returning to the upright position. (You won't of course be able to reach so far forward during the later stages of pregnancy!)

- Repeat 10 to 20 times.

Back Stretch
This stretch complements the previous exercise.
- Lie on your back with your knees bent so that your feet are flat on the floor and slightly apart.
- Stretch your arms back and above your head.
- Keeping your arms relaxed, breathe in, expanding your stomach and arching your back slightly off the floor.
- Then breathe out all your air, pulling the back of your waist into the floor so that your tailbone lifts very slightly, and stretching your arms out backwards as far as you can.
- Repeat 10 to 20 times.

Toning Up

The following tone-up exercises are for the pelvis, abdomen, back, legs, arms, bottom and breasts.

Pelvic Tilt
This exercise is particularly good for relieving backache. It tones up the muscles of the pelvic floor area (the muscles that form a figure 8 around your vagina and anus – crucial during labour) and abdomen.
- Lie flat on the floor with your legs bent, knees together, feet slightly apart and arms by your sides.
- Arch your back slightly, then push the small of your back into the floor and tighten your buttock muscles. As you do this you will feel your tummy muscles gently tighten also.
- Relax.
- Repeat 10 times.

Leg Stretch
You will need to use a chair, mantelpiece or doorknob for support.
- Stand at right angles to your support with your back and

legs straight, feet together.
* Balance your weight on the leg nearest your support and lift the outside leg a few inches from the ground in front of you – or higher if you can – making sure you keep the toes pointed.
* Bend and straighten the knee six times.
* Then turn round and repeat with the other leg.

Bottom Toner
This is an excellent exercise for toning the pelvic area and stomach.
* Lie on the floor with your legs bent, feet apart and arms by your sides.
* Raise your bottom slightly off the floor so that the weight of your body is supported by the upper part of your back.
* Tighten and relax the buttock muscles (this is only a little movement, the hips should not be moving too much). Do it 30 times to start with but try to work up to 100 if you can.

Breast Toner
* Stand straight and hold your left wrist with your right hand and your right wrist with your left hand.
* Keep your wrists away from your body and raise your arms to chin level or higher – the higher the better.
* Clasping your wrists firmly, push towards your elbows as hard as you can in short, sharp movements – 30 times or as many as you can comfortably manage.
* Move your arms up and down as you do this exercise, from chin to eye level.

Upper Arms
* Standing, hold your arms straight out to the sides at right angles to your body.
* Clench your fists to tense the arms.
* Rotate both arms together in small, tight circles – backwards 20 times, then forwards 20 times.

Scissors in the Air

This exercise is very good for the stomach and legs.

- Lie flat on your back and bend your knees up towards your chin.
- Holding on to your thighs, curl the top part of your body forward towards your knees so that your head and shoulders come off the floor.
- Straighten your legs out completely (towards the ceiling); let go of your thighs and stretch your arms to the ceiling.
- You should now be stretching upwards with legs, arms and head.
- Keeping your legs very straight (toes either pointed or flexed towards you) criss-cross them in large, slow scissor movements in the air.
- This is a smooth, sweeping scissor action, don't jerk. Start with 10 and see if you can build up to 50 'scissors'.

Back Arch

This exercise is for the spine, stomach and pelvic area and is another good one for relieving backache.

- Kneel on all fours with your arms straight out beneath you directly in line with your shoulders.
- Breathe out all your air, humping up your back, pulling your stomach in towards your backbone and letting your head drop right forward – try to touch your chest with your chin.
- Then breathe in deeply, pushing your bottom into the air, arching your back and lifting your head up and back so that you can see the ceiling.
- Repeat this whole movement up to 6 times.

Yoga

The yoga positions described here have been designed especially to be safe throughout pregnancy (unless you have a history of miscarriage, in which case it might be best not to attempt them at all. Check with your doctor.)

Mountain Pose
- Stand straight with your feet together. Don't lean over your toes but keep your weight evenly distributed between the balls of your feet and your heels.
- Stretch your whole body up towards the ceiling as though the top of your head was attached to it by a string. Keep your chin down slightly and let your shoulders relax, holding them back and down at the same time.
- Breathe deeply.

Baddha Konasana
- Sit on the floor with your back against a wall and bring the soles and heels of your feet together.
- Catch hold of your toes with your hands, straighten your back, then press your knees downwards towards the floor so that your thighs open wider.
- Hold your legs in this position for as long as you can – try to work the time up from, say, 10 seconds to a few minutes.

Virasana (Hero Pose)
This is a lovely open upward stretch that really feels good as well as being excellent for toning the spine and pelvic area. It also relaxes tired legs.
- Kneel down with your feet on either side of your buttocks, which should be resting on the floor (if necessary, support your bottom with a cushion).
- Make sure your toes are pointing backwards as far as they can so that you feel the stretch along your legs, and keep your back straight.
- Intertwining your fingers, lift your hands above your head and hold for a few minutes.

Squatting
This 'birth' position helps to stretch the muscles of the pelvic floor in preparation for labour. It is most important to practise it right from the beginning of pregnancy until the very end.

- Stand with your feet about 45–60 cm/18–24 in apart, toes pointing slightly outward.
- Crouch down in a squatting position, knees out and your back straight. Try to keep your feet flat on the floor (go onto your toes if you can't manage this at first).
- Hold on to a support (the arms of a low chair, for instance) to begin with, if you need to.
- Stay squatting for about a minute to start with, but try and work up to 5 minutes, and go into it when you can throughout the day.

Savasana (Corpse Pose)
- Lie on your back with your eyes closed (check first that you are lying in a straight line), legs slightly apart and your arms resting at about an angle of 45 degrees to your body, palms upwards.
- Your spine should be flat on the floor – if you find this uncomfortable or difficult, try placing a cushion under your thighs.
- Now, starting with your feet, go through each part of your body slowly tensing and relaxing it (imagine your tension and worries disappearing as you do so).
- Flex your toes up towards you, then relax them.
- Tighten and relax the muscles in your calves, thighs, buttocks and stomach – imagine your stomach touching your backbone.
- Make fists with your hands and relax them, tighten and relax your arms, raise your shoulders and let them sink back, lift your head and let it relax back.
- Screw up your face and relax it, keeping your mouth slightly open so that your jaw is relaxed.
- Having relaxed your body, now concentrate on nice, slow, rhythmical breathing.
- Breathe in, filling your lungs and expanding your stomach, then breathe out, emptying them.
- Continue to lie in this position for as long as you like or have time for. It is a good way to end an exercise session

and is also useful if sleeping becomes difficult in the later months of pregnancy.

Sports

If you are used to regular sporting activities there is no reason why you should not continue through the first half of pregnancy providing everything is progressing normally and your doctor gives you the go-ahead. You only have to use your common sense to know the obvious exceptions: skiing (on snow or water) and horse riding are out (although extremely experienced participants often ignore warnings – members of the Royal family are well-known examples!) Cycling is fine as long as you make sure that you don't tire yourself or lose balance. Stick to quiet roads and cycle paths rather than busy traffic areas. Remember that an accident in early pregnancy could result in miscarriage and that, once your abdomen really grows, the sheer bulk hinders balance and makes anything requiring balance precarious. Better still, perhaps, use an exercise bike in the safety of your own home!

By the latter stages of pregnancy it is unlikely that any blow to the abdomen would actually harm the baby, yet bear in mind that shock might bring on miscarriage or early labour. Apart from monitoring your blood glucose levels carefully before and after sport, diabetes is not the intrusive factor here: all pregnant women are given the same advice as to their limitations as far as sport and exercise go.

Unless there are any complications in your pregnancy there is absolutely no excuse for not walking! Mountaineering, cross-country runs and hiking are not advisable for the amount of strain they will place on you, but replacing short car or bus journeys with a brisk walk can only be beneficial.

Swimming

Swimming is an excellent way of exercising all your muscles. The heavier you feel the more you will appreciate the feeling of weightlessness in the water. Swimming will strengthen your cardiovascular (heart and blood) system and, being an aerobic exercise, it will increase the body's consumption of oxygen. Even if you don't swim you can still do exercises in the water and many public baths and health clubs run aquatic exercise (aquaerobic) classes or even special 'aquanatal' classes for pregnant women (see below).

When swimming always remember:

- Never swim alone in the sea or an empty pool. If you are going to a public pool unaccompanied, tell the lifeguard you have diabetes and ask him or her to keep an eye on you just in case you should become hypo.
- Lower your insulin or have an extra snack before entering the water. Keep glucose tablets handy near the side of the pool or ask the lifeguard to look after them.
- Wear ID, preferably in the form of jewellery or something that you can wear in the pool.
- Don't allow yourself to become out of breath or over-tired.
- Never swim in very cold water as you are more likely to get cramp – this is true for all pregnant women.
- Don't try any high-diving while you are pregnant. Only experienced divers should attempt to dive and then only from heights of 1 m/3 ft or less, as the sudden changes in your blood pressure could affect the baby's circulation.

With the above points taken into account you will be able to enjoy swimming virtually up until the birth, becoming more supple and fit into the bargain.

Here are some simple exercises you can do in the water to help tone up your body:

Leg Warm-Ups
- Stand in the pool at a depth where the water is just below your bust.
- Fold your arms under your breasts to support them and run on the spot. Let the pressure of the water gently massage your legs and get your circulation going.
- Do 30 running steps – or as many as you like without over-tiring yourself.

Water Windmills
This is a good exercise for the shoulder joints.
- Stand in the pool with your shoulders just under the water.
- Keeping your arms straight, rotate the left arm backwards in a full circle six times, as if you were doing the backstroke.
- Repeat with the right arm, then change direction and rotate each arm forwards six times.

Water Cycling
- Stand with your back against the side of the pool
- Stretch out your arms and hold on to the side of the pool to keep you afloat.
- Let your body float out in front of you and 'bicycle' with your legs for as long as you wish – but again, stop well short of sheer exhaustion!

Aquaerobics
Gentle on the body yet toning and good for the circulation, aquaerobics have become quite a craze. Many health clubs and local swimming baths hold classes of exercises performed to music in the shallow end (ask non-swimmers to join in, too)
The body is so well-supported during these water work-outs that you have to take care not to overdo the amount of exercise you take...the water masks the early effects of muscle strain. Tell the instructor you are pregnant (and have diabetes), take it easy and enjoy the fun and freedom.

96

Aquanatal Classes

Many leisure centres (in association with midwives and health visitors) run special 'aquanatal' classes for pregnant women. A midwife organizes and runs the class and the exercises are gentle and geared specifically to pregnant women's needs and abilities. Usually there is also a discussion group afterwards for mums to get to know each other and talk over with the midwife their concerns and feelings about their pregnancy.

Jogging

If you have always been a jogger and are fit and healthy then you may continue until you find it too strenuous or causing you discomfort. However, it would not be sensible to take up jogging if you have never exercised in this way previously.

Remember:
- Test your blood glucose levels before and after jogging.
- Adjust insulin and/or snacks accordingly.
- If you don't have a jogging partner, tell someone who lives with or near you how long you expect to be and which route you are taking.
- Always carry ID.

Tennis, Squash and Other Sports

There is no reason why you should not play tennis until you feel restricted (with your doctor's blessing, of course) but the pace will need to be gentle and the stretching limited. The same goes for badminton.

Squash is a different matter as the game, by its very nature, has to be frenetic and may well prove too vigorous while you are pregnant. Golf is an ideal way of relaxing and getting plenty of open-air exercise, although you should be careful not to exhaust yourself with the very long walks involved. Perhaps 9 holes rather than 18 would be a compromise? Again, the rules of carrying glucose tablets, ID and adjusting insulin and/or snacks apply.

Natural Healthcare and Therapies

There are many 'alternative' and holistic techniques that you may find helpful in the treatment of some minor ailments which occur in pregnancy. You may also find them helpful in relieving stress and tension. As stress is known to raise blood glucose levels, any form of relaxation that has a calming effect on you can only be good. Below are descriptions of a few natural healthcare methods which you might like to try.

Reflexology

This is one method of 'barefoot therapy' which is based on the knowledge that feeling good can be generated from the soles of the feet and the principle that there are reflexes in the feet which relate to all parts of the body. Reflexologists aim to discover physical weakness in various parts of the body through the changing texture of the feet as they work on them. As you have diabetes it is most important that you look after your feet, as over many years diabetes can sometimes lead to nerve damage and loss of sensation in the feet. If you wear ill-fitting shoes that cause corns and bunions or do not notice an injury to your foot, infection may be the result with potentially serious consequences.

You may very well find that reflexology massage, which uses tiny pressure movements, is very sensuous and unwinding. Ongoing reflexology has lasting benefits including helping you to determine whether the sensitivity of your feet is being affected by your diabetes.

Alexander Technique

This is a way of becoming more aware of your balance, posture and movement in your everyday life. Not only does it correct your posture (vital in pregnancy) but it can also cure various complaints which are posture-related (such as backache or even stress-induced headaches). Alexander Technique teaches you to use your body effectively to help you to unwind and reduce the tension in your muscles.

Hydrotherapy

Hydrotherapy uses water as a therapy in itself, in many different ways. The use of showers to speed up a sluggish circulation, steam inhalations to relieve blocked noses (so common in pregnancy), and various forms of baths (the jacuzzi, for example, a hot bubbling tub of (often) mineral-rich water) are all forms of hydrotherapy.

If using a jacuzzi, remember that heat lowers the blood glucose levels so you may need some extra carbohydrate beforehand. All people using jacuzzis are advised to limit a session to 15 minutes and you should be extra careful not to go into a jacuzzi between the time of injecting insulin and eating, as the heat will cause the insulin to be absorbed too quickly and may trigger a hypo.

Aromatherapy

Aromatherapy uses 'essential oils' extracted from different parts of a variety of plants. Used either in their pure, potent form or diluted with a base oil, aromatic oils can be used to calm the nerves, stimulate the digestion, as sedatives or just a fantastic-smelling massage. Most aromatherapists use massage as their treatment yet many oils can be used at home, in the bath or for massage by a partner or yourself. Certain oils are not suitable for use in pregnancy; most are extremely potent and only a few drops should be added to the bathwater. It is advisable to consult a reputable aromatherapist for advice on which oils would be best for you to use.

Feeling and Looking Good

Once the first 12 or so weeks of pregnancy have passed and feelings of nausea and sickness (hopefully!) subside, most women acquire a noticeable bloom to their complexion. This rosy glow is mainly due to extra blood circulating around the body. By the 34th week the amount of blood in the circulation may have increased by as much as 50 per cent and this remains true until after the birth when hormone levels fall and the body reverts to its non-pregnant state.

The condition of the skin nearly always changes for the better during pregnancy. Exactly why is not known; it may be because of all that extra blood flow or simply because eating habits become more sensible. Dry skins tend to produce more oil and become more supple, whereas oily skins may become drier. However, some women find that spots arrive unexpectedly; this is probably due to the action of the hormone progesterone, which increases the activity of the sebaceous glands, thus producing more oil. Make sure you cleanse your skin thoroughly every night and try to eat fresh fruit and vegetables and drink plenty of water (preferably bottled water, which contains less detritus than tap water).

You will notice a rounding of your face as the months go on; plumpness of the cheeks and below the jaw is due to fluid retention and extra fat deposits. If your face becomes significantly swollen then this will be due to some excess fluid retention – but that slight extra fullness helps plump out any lines and wrinkles, making you look younger and healthier. Look after your skin at this time by cleansing well and moisturizing daily.

The condition of your hair will change to some degree – whether for better or for worse. In fact, most women report that their hair becomes thicker, glossier and more manageable during pregnancy. Because the body is producing extra sebum your hair may become a little greasier but the sebum protects its elasticity and prevents the hair from splitting. You may find that you need to wash your hair more often but if you use a mild, frequent-use shampoo you should have a healthy, shining head of hair.

If your hair seems to become drier then you should take extra care to make up for the lack of sebum. Do not brush your hair harshly or use too much heat on it...try to let it dry naturally. Condition it well after every wash. Try to include more fruit and vegetables in your diet...you may be lacking some necessary vitamins if you are not producing the required amount of sebum.

Hair grows much faster during pregnancy than at any other time, but this rapid growth rate will slow down after the birth and some women find that they lose a considerable amount of hair after delivery. If this happens, do not worry...it is a normal occurrence and will not lead to baldness – new hair grows in to replace the hair that has been lost almost immediately.

Getting your hair cut might suit you now, not only to balance the shape of your face (which may have become more rounded) but also to minimize the amount of time you have to fiddle with it, especially if you are working. A style that is easy to manage will serve you well once you have your new baby at home when you are establishing routines of feeding, nappy-changing and so on plus keeping up your diabetes regime. You may feel like a change of colour, though some hairdressers prefer not to use chemical colourants during pregnancy as they believe there is a risk of the dyes entering the bloodstream via a tiny scratch on the scalp. It has not been proved that this could be harmful to the baby but some doctors advise against using hair products that contain potent chemical dyes. Semi-permanent colourants which are based on vegetable dyes might be a good option. There is no evidence that ammonia fumes from a perm could affect the baby, though some doctors might advise you to wait until the first 12 weeks have passed, just to be on the safe side.

Staying Fashionable

Being pregnant certainly does not mean you have to change your style of dress as there are plenty of maternity clothes which are fashionable – and plenty of non-maternity clothes (such as leggings, track bottoms, elasticated skirts, etc.) which can be bought bigger than your normal size to allow for your expanding waistline. There is no way of knowing how large you will eventually be or, indeed, when you will actually show your pregnancy. Some women look pregnant at three to four months whereas others don't until well into their sixth month.

Remember that comfort is all and, although wearing tight clothes will not harm your baby, they will simply serve to make you feel bigger than you really are. Wrap-around skirts, sarongs, undarted shifts, A-line coats and large blouses are all useful items to have in your wardrobe. Avoid clingy fabrics which will show every bulge you possess; where possible choose natural fibres such as cotton and wool rather than man-made ones, which are more likely to make you sweat. Replace elastic in old favourites' waistbands with a drawstring if necessary. Wear low-heeled shoes or trainers which have plenty of room to allow for swollen feet, but not so loose-fitting that they slip off and cause you to fall or develop blisters. Always wear a bra during pregnancy, regardless of whether or not you wore one previously. If you don't, the weight of your growing breasts will stretch the ligaments and you will end up with permanently sagging breasts. As your breast size increases make sure the bra is supportive with wide, adjustable straps; if your breasts feel uncomfortable and heavy at night, sleep in a lightweight version of the same.

Minor Body Changes and Annoying Complaints

However healthy your pregnancy and however good you feel there are a number of bothersome and sometimes uncomfortable symptoms that are extremely common but none the less irritating. Throughout this book we have mentioned various minor complaints such as heartburn, constipation and haemorrhoids. Below are some more:

Bleeding Gums

Pregnancy hormones cause the gums to thicken, soften and swell. They may bleed after brushing the teeth or after eating certain foods and your mouth may feel generally sore. To avoid gingivitis (the name for the condition caused by bacteria building up from food particles trapped in the hollows at the base of the teeth) oral and dental hygiene are essential. Brush your teeth regularly after food, floss and visit the dentist regularly. (Treatment is free while you are pregnant – tell your dentist as soon as you know you are pregnant. He or she will not be able to X-ray your teeth until after the first trimester.)

High blood glucose levels can also lead to gum infections, but providing yours are well controlled this should not be the case.

Cramps

Night-time cramps in the thigh, calf and foot can be very painful. They are thought to be caused by low levels of calcium in the blood, so make sure you are eating enough calcium-rich foods (see Chapter 9 on diet). Rarely, cramps can be caused by a lack of salt in the diet. If you do get cramp, flex your foot and try to massage the affected part firmly and move it around as much as possible.

Backache

Apart from your burgeoning weight, backache can also be a problem during pregnancy because your joints and ligaments are softened by the hormone progesterone. The lower spine

103

takes most of the extra strain and bad posture makes the problem worse. Exercise the spine (see earlier in this chapter) and wear low-heeled, comfortable shoes. Keep your spine straight when standing or sitting and make sure you are not hunched over when driving or sitting down.

Blocked Nose

Pregnant women often suffer from uncomfortable congestion and bleeding, stuffy or runny noses. Nasal discomfort is caused by high levels of pregnancy hormones softening and thickening the mucous membranes in the nose. Dry atmospheres make a stuffy nose worse. Try inhaling Friars Balsam for relief but do not use nasal sprays or drops without consulting your doctor as these can have a rebound effect and make the congestion worse.

Brown Patches on the Skin

The skin around the nipples will darken and you may notice a brown line running down the centre of your abdomen from the lower ribs to the pubic hair. This is called the linea nigra and is quite common in pregnancy; it usually gets darker as the pregnancy progresses. Freckles, some scars, moles and birthmarks often deepen and some women develop a freckly, butterfly-shaped 'mask' across the forehead known as *chloasma*, which is brought out if exposed to the sun. The pattern looks rather like a tea-stain and should be covered by sunblock or shaded with a hat. Darker-haired women are more prone to increased pigmentation.

Stretchmarks

These are thin, red, scar-like lines that occur very suddenly during pregnancy where the skin stretches on the stomach, breasts and thighs. In fact, stretchmarks can occur at any time whether you are pregnant or not if you gain a lot of weight. Some women are more prone to them than others; it probably depends on the elasticity of a woman's skin. They fade to silvery marks but once there, remain for life. Creams and ointments will help keep the skin supple but have little effect on the marks themselves. The only advice can be: watch your weight!

Eye Disturbances

An increase in fluid may cause the shape of the eyeball to change slightly. Sometimes in diabetes there are changes in the lens of the eye if blood glucose levels are badly controlled. See an optician specializing in diabetes to make sure any problem is due to pregnancy and stop wearing contact lenses if they feel at all different.

Pelvic Floor Problems

The enlarging uterus pressing on the bladder may cause leakage of urine at certain times (e.g. when you laugh). A helpful exercise is tensing and relaxing the pelvic floor muscles (as if you were stopping yourself passing urine) as often as you can throughout the day. You can do these while driving, standing, watching TV...anywhere. The more you strengthen these muscles, the less problem you will have with leakages and the stronger they will be for the birth and afterwards.

Varicose Veins

The veins in the leg may dilate and stretch if the strain on them becomes too great. Varicose veins appear as purple lines on the skin which ache and often itch before they become noticeable. Long hours of standing or sitting (especially with your legs crossed) and wearing tight boots, plus hereditary factors can contribute towards varicose veins. Try to put your feet up as often as possible (you'll be glad of the excuse!)

Carpal Tunnel Syndrome

Water retention in the wrists can put pressure on the nerve endings and cause a numbness or loss of feeling in the fingers. Although disconcerting, this condition is not serious and sensitivity returns to the fingers soon after the birth.

Lovemaking

It is certainly possible to enjoy lovemaking during pregnancy. so long as you have no history of miscarriage. Many women claim to feel more sensitive and easily aroused during the middle months, which may be put down to the high levels of hormones circulating in the body, making the breasts and genital organs highly sensitive and extra-responsive. Some women, however, do genuinely 'go off' sex for one reason or another...perhaps they find it distasteful (or their partner does), fear it might harm the baby, feel that they are unattractive and therefore undesirable or simply find lovemaking uncomfortable. But, so long as you have no history of miscarriage, there is no reason why you can't have as full – and possibly more adventurous! – love life as before.

Hopefully you will continue to enjoy an active sex life in the knowledge that it cannot harm your baby (the uterus is completely sealed by a mucous plug) and, assuming you are not going to be *too* athletic (so you don't over-exert yourself or risk injury), he will be completely protected. Early on in pregnancy of course it is particularly important not to be too strenuous, but once the first 12 weeks are up the baby will be completely protected.

Towards the end of your pregnancy there is a possibility that an orgasm could set off contractions strong enough to initiate labour. It has been suggested that the hormone prostaglandin found in the male semen may also bring on labour as this is the same hormone used in the pessaries given to induce it artificially. This, however, is very unlikely as the amount of prostaglandin found in semen is only minute.

Obviously, you may have to adopt positions to accommodate your growing abdomen, but with patience and understanding you and your partner should be able to continue for as long as you wish.

Do remember that blood glucose levels may become low after sex and you should keep glucose tablets by your side. If you know that this happens regularly, a chocolate treat before lovemaking might be a nice idea...

Holidays and Travel

Unless you have had any problems or complications, travelling should be fine unless it involves a particularly arduous journey to somewhere very remote and/or with poor standards of general hygiene. Flying through time zones may upset your routine but you can usually adapt your diabetes regime to fit in. Plane journeys until week 28 are fine but if you really must fly after this time the airline will require you to have a doctor's letter confirming that you are fit to fly and giving the date that the baby is expected.

If you are travelling, don't forget to take:

- Insulin
- Syringes
- Insulin pen
- Testing strips (and meter if you use one)
- Ketone testing strips
- Lancets and pricker
- Log book for blood/urine test results
- Glucagon and/or Hypostop gel
- ID jewellery and/or card
- Glucose tablets, snacks, flask or cool-box
- A letter from your doctor showing that you have diabetes (in case you are stopped at customs and suspected of carrying drugs)
- Form E111 from the DSS (if travelling within the EC)

Some countries do not have U100 insulin (as Britain has) but use U40 instead (which should only be drawn up in U40 syringes). A comparable insulin to the one you use should be available if you should need it. The BDA provide travel leaflets covering many countries (see Useful Addresses). It's a good idea when travelling to take twice as much of everything and, even if you use a pen injector, take some syringes in case the pen happens to break. Always carry equipment in your hand luggage, never put it in the hold of the plane as it will freeze. If you are travelling with someone else it would be as well to let him or her carry some of what you will need in case your bag gets lost or stolen. If you are travelling alone, split the equipment up between two bags, or between a jacket pocket/bumbag and, say, a small hold-all that you can use as hand luggage.

Don't be fazed by long-haul flights. It may be uncomfortable sitting there with your tummy pressed against the pull-down food tray, but once you arrive you'll forget the journey. Insulin injections can be fitted in depending on the length of the flight and the time difference. If you have, say, an eight-hour flight to Florida (remember, the day you travel will be five hours longer for you because that part of the US is five hours behind the UK) you may need an extra dose of short-acting insulin on the plane to cope with having extra meals. Make sure you eat regularly and test your blood glucose frequently during the flight to keep things under control.

If you are going to a hot country, remember that the heat can affect your absorption of insulin and make your blood glucose levels drop. Do blood tests and adjust your insulin to allow for this. Also, reduce insulin or eat extra snacks if you are planning on doing lots of swimming. After the first few days you will see a pattern emerging which you can stick to until you return home.

Pets and Pregnancy

While you are pregnant, make sure you always wash your hands after handling cats and kittens, however clean they seem. Cat faeces contain *Toxoplasma gondii*, an organism that causes *Toxoplasmosis* (which may lead to a range of problems in the unborn baby). If you have a cat, of course the cat litter tray must be cleaned out, but if possible you should get someone else to do the job and remove the soiled litter from the tray. If you have to do this yourself, either wear light disposable gloves or use ordinary gloves and wash them and your hands afterwards. (incidentally, raw meat contains this organism as well, which will be discussed in Chapter 9). Always wear gloves while gardening in case the soil has been fouled by cats. Make sure dogs and cats are wormed regularly and always use separate utensils for their meals.

A HEALTHY DIET FOR YOU AND YOUR BABY

Diet Myths Exploded

Diabetes and pregnancy – each has a widely-held dietary myth attached to it:

- People with diabetes are on a special diet and can never eat sugar.
- An expectant mother should 'eat for two'.

As you will see (or already know), there is no such thing these days as a 'diabetic diet'; this is probably the most misunderstood subject concerning diabetes. The eating plan given to people with diabetes is that which is recommended for the general population: high-fibre, low-fat, low-sugar with plenty of starchy carbohydrate.

As far as 'eating for two' goes, this is an old-fashioned dictum that went out with post-war rationing! Eating a well-balanced, healthy diet will ensure that you and your baby get the nutrients you need. Eating for two is simply over-eating and will result in you putting on far too much weight, high blood glucose levels and the nearly impossible task of losing kilos of fat after the birth. It is very important to balance the amount of food you eat to your insulin requirements – if your diet is erratic this will cause erratic blood glucose levels – your dietitian will help you work out the quantities of food you need.

How Dietary Thinking Has Changed

As mentioned earlier, in pre-insulin days there was little question of diet...the only diet that would help someone with diabetes stay alive for any length of time was virtual starvation
with the prospect of boiled cabbage as a daily treat. Indeed,
one German physician at the beginning of this century recommended one complete day of fasting (known as 'metabolic
Sunday') each week.

When insulin first came into use it was assumed that both
types of carbohydrates (sugary and starchy) were detrimental to
diabetes and these were virtually banned. The foods that
someone with diabetes was advised to eat and fill up with were
mainly those containing plenty of fat and protein; carbohydrate intake was kept at a strictly measured minimum.
However, people with diabetes do have a higher-than-average
chance of developing heart disease and this would not have
been helped by the high fat intake.

An invaluable lesson had been learned by as long ago as the
Second World War: fibre was found to have beneficial attrib-
utes for everybody. It was also noted that foods containing
fibre helped fill an empty stomach more successfully than those
that had been refined (obviously important in the days of
rationing). Between 1941 and 1954 high-fibre National Flour
was in compulsory use in the UK, and it was found that even
though sugar consumption was higher during the early 1950s
than before the War, the death rate from diabetes fell dramatically. One enlightened doctor, Hugh Trowell, offered the theory that it was the lack of fibre rather than the sugar in the diabetic diet which could be of great importance in controlling
blood glucose levels. But if people with diabetes continued to
keep their consumption of carbohydrate low, they would not
be able to include anything like enough fibre in their diet as

111

this 'roughage' (the part of the food that is not digested) is only to be found in foods containing carbohydrate. Indeed, some carbohydrates contain a particularly high percentage of soluble fibre (pulses, beans, peas, lentils, oats and some fruits).

After exhaustive trials it was found that these soluble fibres actually slowed down the absorption of sugar (and fat lipids) into the bloodstream and helped keep blood glucose levels under control. Fibre was also found necessary for the healthy functioning of the bowel and seen to reduce the risk of developing disorders such as cancer of the bowel, diverticulitis and haemorrhoids. Once the great importance of fibre had been proven it became rather obvious that many – often fatal – diseases could have been prevented by the diet which is now recommended to the whole population, including to those with diabetes.

Diet Over the Last Two Decades

Once research showed that a drastic reassessment of diet should be made for the general population (and that included people with diabetes) new UK governmental guidelines spawned plenty of trendy slimming regimes based on high-fibre, low-fat recipes. Along with this revolution – which made cholesterol a dirty word – came new products to help weight-watchers everywhere. Although saccharine has been available since – believe it or not – the last century, the advent of a wider variety of artificial sweeteners was one major answer to the slimmer's prayer. In turn, those grappling with the tedious regime of an old-fashioned diabetic diet benefited beyond their wildest dreams.

Rita, now 50, remembers:

Being diabetic in the sixties was, not to put too fine a point on it, quite loathsome as I recall. I ate eggs, cheese and red meat until I couldn't stand the sight of anything I was given. My diet in the last 15 years or so has mainly been based on pasta...I still can't believe that I'm actually allowed to have it!

In fact, pasta, potatoes, pulses, bread and vegetables are now heartily recommended for those with diabetes, and with so many unrefined wholemeal and wholewheat varieties around there's a superb choice. Small amounts of sucrose (ordinary table sugar) may be used in baking, and dessert treats can be eaten at the end of a high-fibre meal. If you haven't already noticed, 'lite', low or sugar-free substitutes are available for almost every kind of sweet food or drink now available. Most nutritional food values are clearly detailed on product packaging. Some people with diabetes still weigh their portions of food, but since nutritional labelling has become the norm this is unnecessary as you will be able to tell at a glance what the carbohydrate and fat content of a single item is.

Although some pregnant women who have diabetes are given a certain daily carbohydrate allowance, this is used as a flexible guideline. You should also watch your fat intake to avoid putting on unnecessary weight.

Carbohydrates Explained

Although the role of carbohydrates (CHO) in the management of diabetes has changed, it is the food group that directly affects blood glucose and so is of the greatest significance to you. Carbohydrates provide energy and are extremely important to our health (so long as they are not the fast-acting, sugary variety).

There are two main types of carbohydrates: starchy and sugary.

Starchy Carbohydrates
The main sources are of starch are:

- bread
- cereals (wheat, oats, corn, barley, etc.)

- rice
- potatoes
- pulses (beans and lentils)
- cereal-based products (including biscuits)

Fruit and vegetables contain some starchy carbohydrate but also contain their own sugars. However, their sugar content is small and is tied up with fibre so it is more slowly absorbed into the bloodstream than 'straight' sugar would be.

Sugary Carbohydrates

Sugar, honey, jam, chocolates, sweet biscuits, tinned fruit in syrup, sweetened drinks...no one needs these foods to keep healthy – in fact they have the opposite effect, giving rise to obesity and tooth decay.

Apart from these foods being absorbed straight into the bloodstream and raising the blood glucose levels rapidly they are simply bad for you – unless, of course, you are in a hypo situation. There are so many sugar-free alternatives on the market it is difficult to see why anyone would resort to the 'real thing'. However, a little bit of what you fancy (and it's usually chocolate for most people) won't hurt after a high-fibre meal and may be essential before exercise.

Diabetic Products

With modern artificial sweeteners being used in many slimming and health products now, plus the realization that small amounts of ordinary sugar do little harm, special diabetic products have no place in today's diet. These products are expensive and include high quantities of fat and flour to make them more palatable so are just as fattening as their ordinary counterparts. Far better to go for pure fruit spreads or low-sugar jams. Also look for jellies, yoghurts and drinks containing

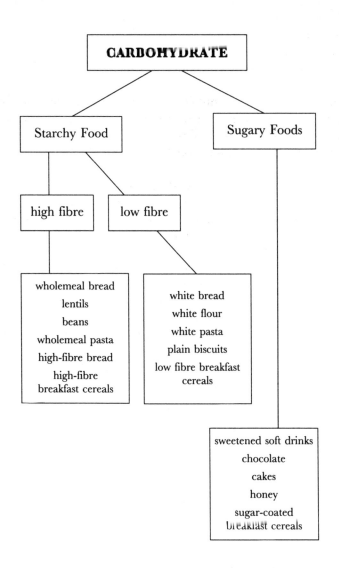

Carbohydrates at a glance

the artificial sweeteners saccharine, Aspartame and Acesulphame potassium.

A Balanced Diet

Try to keep a good balance of essential protein, minerals and vitamins in your diet. You can make sure you are getting all the necessary nutrients by planning your daily meals from the four basic groups:

1. Dairy products
2. Bread and cereals
3. Vegetables and fruit
4. Meat, fish and eggs

Within the four groups listed are plenty of foods you will be able to enjoy while avoiding those high in sugar, fat and unrefined carbohydrates.

Dairy Products

Milk is a most useful dairy product in pregnancy as it is high in both protein and calcium. You should try to have a pint a day, but as whole milk is rich in fat it would be preferable to use skimmed or semi-skimmed varieties as these contain the same amount of calcium as whole milk but less fat. Never drink unpasteurized cow's or goat's milk during pregnancy as it has not been sterilized. If you find it difficult to drink as much as a pint of milk in a day, 1 oz of low-fat cheese (such as Edam, Gouda or low-fat cheddar) or a small carton of yoghurt contains the same amount of calcium as one third of a pint of milk. Using low-fat yoghurt, fromage frais and cheese will help keep down your fat intake (but see information on Listeria later in this chapter). A small portion of ice-cream is rich in

116

calcium, so a low-sugar brand would make an ideal dessert. Natural yoghurt or fromage frais makes a good dessert substitute for cream, which is high in fat.

If you are under 18 your dietitian may suggest extra calcium as requirements for this age group are higher.

Bread and Cereals

Breakfast cereals that contain the whole grain (oat, wheat, corn, etc.) are perfect high-fibre sources of carbohydrate, as is wholemeal bread (or white bread containing oat fibre). Use wholemeal pasta, rice and pizza bases wherever possible. Wholemeal flour has been known to turn some people's recipes into soggy disasters, however, so if you're not confident about your baking prowess use half white and half wholemeal. Always look out for wholemeal or wholewheat labels on biscuits and cereals; *neither* **wheatmeal** nor **wheatgerm** is a high-fibre product and this can be confusing. Cereal bars with fruit make perfect snacks.

Vegetables and Fruit

All vegetables are excellent sources of vitamins and minerals. They are best eaten raw or steamed to avoid loss of nutrients during cooking, although they can also be boiled in a small amount of water for a short period of time (blanched) without too great a loss. Potatoes in particular are also a good source of fibre (especially jacket potatoes or any recipe that includes the skin). Sliced potato skins are a much healthier alternative to chips, which are very fatty. If you must have chips occasionally, the reduced-fat oven-ready or microwaveable varieties are a slightly lesser evil than those you fry. Mashed potatoes contain less fibre than those baked in their jackets but are still a good source of vitamins and minerals.

Citrus fruits are particularly high in vitamin content. Try not to eat large quantities of mangoes and grapes as these are high in their own sugar (fructose). Bananas are delicious, not fattening and full of fibre. Dried fruit such as raisins, sultanas and dates contain their own concentrated sugars but can be used in small quantities, for instance to sweeten cereals.

Some fruits – such as strawberries, blackberries, raspberries and rhubarb – are very low in (sugary) carbohydrate and can be eaten freely; they make good desserts.

Meat, Fish and Eggs

This group is an excellent source of protein. Red meats and offal contain plenty of iron – although pregnant women are recommended to avoid liver as its high levels of Vitamin A may be poisonous to the baby.

Try and make cuts of meat as lean as possible; remove the skin from chicken as it is very fatty. White fish (cod, haddock, halibut, sole, etc.) have similar nutritional values to poultry. Small-boned tinned fish such as pilchards, sardines, tuna and herring are rich in calcium, iron and protein.

Other Essential Nutrients for a Healthy Pregnancy

Planning your meals and snacks sensibly throughout the day (your dietitian can help you) will ensure that you and your baby get all the nutrients, vitamins and minerals you need. Protein, calcium and iron are important because:

- calcium helps in the development of your baby's teeth and bones
- protein is tissue-building and essential for your baby's growth, a healthy placenta and uterus
- iron increases the number of red cells in the blood and will help to prevent you becoming anaemic (as your blood

increases in volume and tends to thin). If you are found to be anaemic your doctor may prescribe iron tablets to supplement your diet.

You also need enough of the following to ensure a healthy pregnancy:

Fats and Oils

Try to avoid saturated fats such as butter. Choose spreads or cooking oils containing polyunsaturated fatty acids (corn and sunflower oil) or monounsaturated fatty acids (olive, rapeseed or peanut oil).

Folic Acid

Helps fight anaemia and helps prevent neural tube defects in the baby. It can be found in, raw, dark green leafy vegetables such as spinach, pulses, wholemeal bread, oranges and bananas.

If you are suffering from a deficiency of folic acid you may be prescribed supplements in tablet form.

B Vitamins

Essential for a healthy skin, mental stability and for the correct functioning of the digestive system. After the birth they increase the production of milk for breastfeeding. You can find B vitamins in, meat, eggs, wholemeal bread, wheatgerm, fish and yeast extract.

Vitamin C

Helps the body absorb iron and keep tissues strong and healthy. Citrus fruits and green vegetables contain Vitamin C.

Vitamin D

Helps the body maintain the level of calcium and phosphorus in the blood. Main sources are, fatty fish, eggs, butter and margarine.

It is also produced when the body is exposed to sunlight.

Vitamin E

Can help strengthen the foetus and placenta and improve the circulation, thus helping to prevent varicose veins and haemorrhoids. Good sources include, eggs, dairy products, unpolished (unrefined) rice, wholemeal bread, and vegetable oils.

You can take vitamin E as wheatgerm oil in supplement form but you should never take vitamin E along with iron, as iron destroys vitamin E's effectiveness. To avoid this, leave a 12-hour gap between taking either supplement.

Zinc

Important for healthy cell walls and for the effectiveness of enzymes working in your body. Zinc is present in, milk, vegetables, meat, fish, and sunflower seeds.

Fluids

Fluids are an important part of your diet and you should try to drink two pints of liquid a day. Always use diet drinks unless you are feeling hypo. Pure fruit juices are concentrated and high in their own sugar so it is recommended that they are taken with meals rather than used as thirst-quenchers. Plenty of water (preferably bottled) is a good idea especially if you are overweight (no calories and it helps to clear out your system) – helps clear the complexion, too.

Having diabetes, you will be used to watching your alcohol consumption carefully – but you must be extra-aware in pregnancy. Not only does alcohol lower the blood glucose but there is some concern that excess alcohol may harm the baby. Drink in moderation or, if you can, avoid it altogether.

Vegetarians and Vegans

If you follow a vegetarian diet, take extra care that you are getting enough protein daily. For vegetarians, eggs and dairy products are prime sources of protein. Vegans should eat plenty of dried fruits, pulses, nuts and seeds, wholemeal bread, pasta and cereals.

If you do not eat dairy produce, make a real effort to find as many protein-enriched substitutes as possible. Soya beans are perfect and there are many soya products on the market: soya milk, soya flour and soya 'meat' (known as *tofu*). It is also advisable to take vitamin-B supplements since these vitamins – B_{12} in particular – are found mainly in animal foods. Yeast extract is a good source.

Vegetarians and vegans – indeed anyone on a specialized diet – should take advice from the dietitian at the diabetes clinic.

Looking After Your Weight

As we have already pointed out, anyone who suggests you should be 'eating for two' should be politely ignored. A well-balanced diet is important throughout everyone's life but never more so than during pregnancy and especially if you have diabetes. As your pregnancy progresses your insulin requirements will become far higher than normal, which will mean you must eat wisely and well. Your carbohydrate intake may need to be adjusted and re-distributed throughout pregnancy to match your insulin intake and individual appetite. It is not healthy for anyone to be overweight (or underweight, for that matter) and a large weight-gain during pregnancy could give rise to high blood pressure, swelling of the feet and ankles and undue strain on the heart – not to mention the havoc that being overweight will play on your blood glucose levels (your insulin will not work so efficiently). Granted, the mother-to-be with diabetes has to tread a very fine line, all things considered, but many doctors and nurses will agree that the best controlled person with diabetes is the one who is pregnant. The realization of how much is at stake certainly comes home to you at this time more than ever.

Your weight will be watched keenly during pregnancy. You may be weighed every time you attend clinic; if you seem to be putting on too much weight too early in the pregnancy you will certainly be advised on how to cut down sensibly for a steady weight gain (not weight loss). If necessary, a diet plan may be made taking in your day-to-day requirements.

On average, a woman on a well-balanced diet will put on around 11 to 12.5 kg/25 to 30 lb during pregnancy (some put on a lot more or slightly less than this). The gain is due to the combined weight of the baby, placenta, increasing blood supply to the uterus (at full term the uterus takes about 25 per cent of the body's blood supply to nourish the baby), amniotic fluid around the baby, water retention plus a natural increase in fat reserves and the enlargement of various organs such as the breasts and the uterus.

Having your own scales at home will help, although you must not panic at every tiny increase. So long as you are doing your best with your diet, regular visits to the clinic should help sort out any problems. Usually unrefined carbohydrates and foods high in fat and protein are the calorie-laden culprits. Your calorie (energy) needs during pregnancy increase very little, if at all... However, if you do need some extra energy it should only be about 200 extra calories – roughly equivalent to three slices of wholemeal bread – so heavy bingeing sessions are *not* in order!

Heartburn and Indigestion

You are bound to suffer from heartburn and indigestion at some time during your pregnancy; this usually happens after the 30th week when acidity is forced up into the gullet by the enlarging uterus. If this happens you will feel a burning sensation after eating and the more you eat the worse you will feel. Avoid large meals (particularly before bed), fried or spicy food, alcohol, orange juice or coffee. In fact, avoid anything that personally gives you discomfort. Chew your food thoroughly but try to change your daily meal and snack plan by redistributing your carbohydrate into smaller meals throughout the day so that your stomach is never completely empty. Try sucking strong minty sweets (you can buy sugar-free varieties) or consult your doctor, who may prescribe an antacid mixture. Some women find that a small glass of milk (warm if preferred) helps considerably.

Constipation

You will be more prone to constipation during pregnancy, as the hormone that relaxes ligaments and muscles during this time also tends to relax the muscles that control the bowel. If you are keeping to a diet that is high in fibre this problem will be helped considerably. A good fluid intake will also help. However, if you are troubled by constipation, do not take laxatives – they can give you diarrhoea and upset your stomach. Speak to your doctor, who will probably recommend an alkali preparation or senna derivative if he or she feels it necessary. Although it would be ideal to open the bowels daily, it's not imperative so long as you always spare the time when Nature calls. Many sufferers make the situation worse by hurrying and straining, which invariably results in haemorrhoids.

How to Combat Nausea

It is possible to alleviate nausea and sickness by eating frequent snacks of bland, starchy foods such as plain biscuits, dry crackers and toast: indeed, have anything you find helps. Having diabetes, you will be used to your regular snack-times – though you may find that an extra starchy snack (such as a couple of biscuits) before getting out of bed will calm things down considerably. Here are a few hints:

- Keep a store of plain biscuits by your bed for the morning and in case you feel queasy (or hypo) during the night.
- Avoid spreading too much butter (or butter substitute) on toast or bread.
- Warm, milky drinks may make you feel nauseous. Cold drinks are more thirst-quenching.
- Avoid any smell that upsets you: brewing coffee and the greasy smell of frying are common irritants.
- Make sure you eat regularly even if you have lost your appetite. If you are being sick a lot and sometimes cannot manage solids, take your carbohydrates as fluids (your dietitian will suggest alternatives).
- Avoid spicy and creamy foods.

With experience of two pregnancies fraught with nausea, one woman told us:

I went off meat completely. There was no question of a Sunday roast for months on end in our house. My husband had to cook and serve up our meals as I would feel bilious if I could smell anything cooking. I found that absolutely plain pasta with no sauce whatsoever helped a great deal. Plain biscuits helped stave off the nausea, too.

Another recalls:

I banned my husband from eating fried eggs in the house for nine months...yuk!

Cravings

We've all heard stories of pregnant women craving bizarre foods (or worse, eating soil or coal!). This strong desire for unusual foods is called 'Pica' (from the Latin word for magpie, a bird that collects strange things). It is true that pregnant women can be extremely unpredictable in their choice of food – especially during the first three months. Tastes alter when you are pregnant because of the hormonal, metabolic and chemical changes going on in your body.

Some women have strong cravings for foods that they never liked before their pregnancy (or in the case of those with diabetes, are not supposed to have in large amounts!). But true Pica (when a woman is found eating coal or chalk) is most uncommon today – perhaps because most people are more nutritionally aware and iron and vitamin tablets are easily available (though the link between Pica and nutritional deficiency has not been conclusively proven).

There are some foods that are high in certain sources of nourishment so are probably good for you should you develop a sudden desperation for them (if the food you crave is not mentioned in our lists of those high in nutrients, above, check its value out with your dietitian).

Most food obsessions that pregnant women get are short-lived and their attraction is quite likely to be psychological. If you have an uncontrollable urge to eat a slice of gooey rich cake or a cream bun, best to give in to it – the chances are you won't fancy it again. Try to eat it at the end of a high-fibre meal, though! However, if a sweet craving is becoming a regular occurrence, you must try to substitute it with artificially sweetened alternatives (diet chocolate mousse has saved many a desperate chocoholic).

For some reason I wanted to eat ice cubes throughout, each time. My children, David and Laura, crunch away on them to this day!

Mashed potatoes and frozen peas...nearly every meal until the last two months.

Peanuts and peanut butter...but I can't touch them now.

Foods to Avoid

You may have heard about *Listeriosis*. This is an illness caused by *Listeria monocytogenes*, a bacteria found in some foods. Although it is quite rare, Listeria has attracted a certain amount of publicity over the last few years because it appears to be on the increase.

Small quantities of this bacteria do not cause problems for most people; it is only when the bacteria has had a chance to grow to large numbers in food before it is eaten that there is a risk of Listeriosis. Although the symptoms are usually little more than a mild flu-like illness, for a pregnant woman the implications are serious: miscarriage, stillbirth or possible brain damage to the baby.

Because the illness itself is so mild, Listeriosis can be difficult to detect. It is best to avoid the risk by not eating certain foods, and by storing and cooking your food correctly.

Listeria cannot grow in many of the foods we usually keep in the fridge. Some dairy foods can be a problem but, providing you keep your refrigerator temperature really cold (below 3°C/37°F) you only need to avoid the foods listed opposite. Hard white cheeses such as cheddar, Edam, etc. are safe, but remove any rind first. Processed cheeses, yoghurt, cottage cheese and fromage frais sold in sealed containers are all safe.

DON'T EAT:

- Soft ripened cheeses such as Brie and Camembert
- Blue-veined cheeses such as Danish Blue and Stilton
- Any patés; liver sausage, liver paté, etc.
- Raw or undercooked poultry or any meat products.
- Any meat which is still pink or 'blue' should be avoided.
- Unwrapped foods eaten without reheating...i.e., sold loose from a chiller cabinet: cold meats, sausage rolls, quiche, chicken, etc.
- Uncooked foods eaten without first having to be reheated, such as ready-prepared salads, coleslaw, chopped salad ingredients.

Other Cooking and Storing Tips

- If you use a microwave oven, follow cooking instructions to the last letter including standing times and stirring instructions. It is vital that food reaches 70°C/158°F all the way through for two minutes.
- Only reheat leftover foods once.
- Frozen foods are safe if they are correctly thawed and cooked promptly right through.
- Canning destroys Listeria, so tinned foods are safe when they have just been opened. Store leftovers in the fridge (but not still in the tin), eat within five days and only re-heat once.
- Never eat foods which have passed their 'sell by', 'eat by' or 'best before' date, and only eat chilled food on the day of purchase.
- Take-aways can be suspect...food must be piping hot when it reaches you. The same goes for a meals you eat in restaurants.
- It is very unlikely that Listeria can be passed on to your baby by breastmilk, and breastfeeding mothers are at

much lower risk of Listeriosis than when they were pregnant.

- Make sure that cook-chill foods, particularly, are cooked right through and served piping hot.

Avoiding Salmonella

You have also doubtless heard about salmonella poisoning and how this is particularly associated with eggs and poultry. Salmonella is not actually harmful to the baby but is most uncomfortable for the mother! Eggs have certainly attracted bad publicity in recent years yet they are a good source of protein and thus beneficial to your diet. However, we have all been advised not to eat raw eggs or foods with uncooked egg in them. Pregnant women are also advised to eat only eggs which are cooked until both the white and the yolk are solid. If you are following a recipe which requires eggs to be only partially cooked or not cooked at all, use pasteurized egg products (in liquid or dry form) which can be brought in many food shops and supermarkets.

Do take special care when handling raw poultry (and other meats for that matter); always wash your hands before and after preparing food. A meat thermometer is useful to ensure that roasts, etc. are cooked thoroughly.

When storing food, wrap it in foil or clingfilm to stop bacteria spreading from one food to another. Raw meat should never be in contact with cooked meat, for example.

Please don't become over-anxious about the possibility of catching food-related infections – most are very rare and it is unlikely that you or your baby would be affected. However, it is sensible to follow the above advice and take precautions to reduce any risk, however small.

Recipes from the BDA

The BDA have kindly given us some of their recommended recipes which are particularly useful in pregnancy and quite delicious for the rest of the family. Bear in mind that your dietitian can recommend many other dishes as well.

Chicken Stir Fry
Serves 2

1 tblsp/15 ml olive or sunflower oil
1 boneless chicken breast, skin removed, cut into strips
4 spring onions, chopped
1 green pepper, de-seeded and cut into pieces
1 oz/25 g unsalted cashew nuts
4 oz/100 g beansprouts
2 tblsp/30 ml light soy sauce

- Heat oil and stir chicken for 5 minutes or until cooked.
- Add onion, green pepper and nuts and fry for a few minutes.
- Stir in the beansprouts and soy sauce and cook for a further
- 2–3 minutes.
- Serve immediately.

Trout with Almonds
Serves 2

2 trout (approx. 6 oz/175 g each), cleaned and boned
1 tblsp/15 ml low-fat spread
Freshly ground black pepper to taste
½ oz/15 g flaked almonds
Parsley sprig to garnish

- Place the fish on a grill rack. Dot with low-fat spread. Season
- to taste.
- Grill on medium flame/heat, turning occasionally until fish
- flakes easily when tested with a fork.
- Sprinkle with the flaked almonds. Garnish with parsley.
- Serve immediately.

Courgette and Sweetcorn Flan
Serves 6–8

Pastry:
4 oz/100 g wholemeal flour
2 oz/50 g plain flour
2 oz/50 g low-fat spread
1 oz/25 g white vegetable fat
cold water as needed
Filling:
1 medium courgette, sliced
3 oz/75 g sweetcorn
2 oz/50 g reduced fat Cheddar cheese, grated
2 size-3 eggs, beaten
¼ pint/150 ml skimmed milk

- Make the pastry by rubbing the fat into the flour. Knead to a smooth dough with enough water to bind.
- Line an 8-in/20 cm flan ring with the dough.
- Place in the fridge for 15–20 minutes.
- Bake blind (no filling in it) in pre-heated oven at 200°C/400°F/Gas Mark 6 for 10 minutes.
- Remove from oven.

- Place courgette slices, sweetcorn and cheese in flan base.
- Mix eggs and milk. Pour over vegetables.
- Bake at 180°C/350°F/Gas Mark 4 for 35 minutes or until springy to the touch.

Apple Delight
Serves 2

5 oz/150 g carton low-fat natural yoghurt
1 eating apple, peeled, cored and grated
2 tsp/10 ml lemon juice
artificial sweetener to taste (optional)
2 walnut halves

- Place yoghurt in a bowl. Stir in the grated apple and lemon juice. Add sweetener to taste.
- Pile into 2 individual dishes. Chill before serving.
- Top each with a walnut half.

Macaroni Mince
Serves 2–3

8 oz/225 g extra lean minced beef
1 medium onion, finely chopped
1 clove garlic, crushed
1 medium carrot, finely diced
8-oz/225-g can tomatoes
Salt and pepper to taste
Pinch of mixed herbs
2 oz/50 g wholewheat macaroni, or pasta, cooked
1 oz/25 g reduced fat cheddar cheese, grated

- Place minced beef, onion, garlic and carrot in a large pan. Fry until browned, stirring occasionally. (If using a non-stick pan there is no need to use extra oil when browning the meat).
- Stir in the tomatoes, seasonings and herbs, bring to the boil and simmer for 20 minutes.
- Once cooked, place half the mince mixture into an oven-proof dish, layer with the macaroni.
- Place remaining mince over the macaroni. Top with grated cheese.
- Brown under the grill and serve hot.

Nut Roast
Slices to serve 6

1 onion, finely chopped
1 tblsp/15 ml olive or sunflover oil
8 oz/225 g mixed nuts, chopped
4 oz/100 g wholemeal breadcrumbs (reserve 1 tblsp/15 ml)
½ pint/275 ml vegetable stock
2 tsp/10 ml yeast extract
Pinch of mixed herbs
Salt and freshly ground pepper
Tomatoes to garnish

- Sauté the onion in the oil until transparent.
- In a large bowl, combine all the ingredients and mix well. (Should be a slack mixture.)
- Turn into a lightly greased 1-lb/450-g loaf tin and sprinkle with the remaining breadcrumbs.
- Bake at 180°C/350°F/Gas Mark 4 for 30 minutes or until golden brown.
- Allow to cool before turning out.
- Garnish with sliced tomatoes.

Chapter 10

GETTING READY FOR YOUR NEW BABY

Good Planning Is Essential!

Once you have given up work (certainly by week 36 of your pregnancy) you should be getting the household as organized as is humanly possible so that when you bring home your new baby everything is there in a logical place. What you don't want to be doing is scouring the house for a missing article as your new baby screams wildly in the background. The key to a smooth-running household is order – and if that sounds boring to those who prefer living in a chaotic muddle ... be warned!

In fact, the majority of people with diabetes already know how to be organized and keep to a schedule, know where things are and generally keep to a routine: the fact is, they have to. So it should follow that one can apply this same knowledge to organizing the household and preparing to make life as smooth as possible once the baby arrives. The baby is going to tie you down to a schedule, but then so (to an extent) does your diabetes. If you can manage to have the home running smoothly you will find it easier to get into two routines and somehow fit them in with each other.

If you haven't previously been working out of the home – perhaps you already look after your other children full-time – you may well not have acknowledged that now is the time to get a grip on things. The natural hiatus that occurs when you give up work tends to propel you into activity. On the other hand, you may feel tired and in real need of rest. However you feel – energized or lethargic – remember that there's not long to go and there's always a chance that the baby could arrive early...

Organizing the Household

Housework and shopping are going to become more difficult towards the end of pregnancy, so the earlier you start doing big shopping trips for essentials which you can store, so much the better. Clear out a cupboard, spare-room or cellar for tinned and dry goods. Soap, toothpaste, toilet paper, cleaning materials, pet food and so on can be stored indefinitely (so long as the storage place is not damp). Do as many big shopping trips to the supermarket or cash-and-carry as you can manage – imagine you are stocking up for World War Three...that's how life will feel once you arrive home with the baby!

A freezer is a real bonus as you can fill it during the last month of pregnancy with enough provisions to see you through until some time after the birth. If you are unable to drive a car, ask your partner or a relative or friend to help out. Failing this, quite a number of shops, cash-and-carrys and even some supermarkets offer a delivery service. Find out if a local branch does this and ask for delivery charges. You will find that delivery is often free if the order is, say, over £50.

Remember that carrying heavy bags of shopping will put you under strain. Never bend from the waist when picking up heavy weights – bend from the knees and keep your back straight.

Stock Up on Diabetes Equipment

Now is also the time to see your doctor and arrange to have prescriptions dispensed so that your supplies of insulin, blood-test strips and so on will last for several months after the baby has been born. If you have a six-month supply of everything you could possibly need then you will not be caught out at the most inconvenient moment. Take heed of Sandra's experience:

I had completely neglected my insulin supply and, knowing I had enough to cover my eventual hospital stay, put it to the back of my mind. There seemed to be so many other things to organize. Three days after arriving home with the baby I went to refill my insulin pen, looked in the fridge and – you've guessed – no insulin in any shape or form. My injection was due, my husband was out, the baby was tucked up in bed and it was nearly 5 o'clock in the after-noon (when the chemist shuts). I couldn't believe that I'd been so stupid! I had muddled through not really checking how much was in the fridge, just grabbing without looking. I had to get Alexandra out of bed and put her in the car (on a winter's evening) and drive five miles. All I can say is, cover your every need for several months after the birth, by which time you will feel compos mentis enough to realize that you need to re-stock before you get into trouble.

Remember to Stock Up On

- Insulin
- Syringes (if you use them or in case your pen should break)
- Blood-test/urine-test strips
- Hypostop/glucagon
- Ketone-testing strips
- Glucose tablets

The use-by date is usually well ahead of the date of purchase, but before you leave the pharmacy or chemist do check that your supplies have plenty of shelf-life left. If your doctor or pharmacist should query why you need such a large supply on one prescription rather than small amounts with repeat prescriptions, explain that you are going to have enough on your mind and would rather be safe than sorry.

Housework and Daily Chores

If you can afford it, and are lucky enough to find one, someone who will come in for two or three hours a week to give the house a real clean is the best luxury available. If you do look to employ someone, choose a person who could be relied on to keep an eye on the baby so you can have some time for yourself to do some shopping or simply relax.

Most people, however, are not able to indulge in such extravagances and the chances are that the household chores will be down to you (even if you have a partner or relative who is willing to help out some of the time). Try to tidy up as you go along and keep everything free from clutter. Set yourself a couple of mornings a week for housework but resist doing anything that involves physical exertion. You are going to feel pretty exhausted towards the end of your pregnancy and should try to put things into perspective. Neglect anything that is not essential. It's important to keep the house (especially the kitchen) clean but not to the point where you are knocking yourself out. Climbing up and down stairs with a vacuum cleaner is asking for trouble as you become bigger. If there's no one to help, only do this when absolutely necessary. Ask people to take their shoes off when they come in the house, you'll be surprised at the lack of debris! Keeping work surfaces and shelves tidy is the easiest way to make a room look clean. A quick wipe over with a damp cloth from time to time will keep the dust down considerably. Remember also that housework uses up energy, so take that into account and try to do it, say, straight after breakfast when you have just eaten and are unlikely to have low blood glucose levels or feel hypo.

A washing machine is an obvious bonus. Many people without children don't think about buying one until their first baby comes along. If this is the case, take delivery a couple of months before the baby is due so you can get used to the machine and sort out teething problems (if any). It is also possible to hire a washing machine in the same way as you can hire a television, usually from the same kind of rental shop. They are fairly inexpensive on a monthly basis and would tide you over for several months if you were unable to afford to buy one outright.

It's amazing how much washing a tiny baby generates, even if you do use disposable nappies! Ironing can be relaxing though it certainly won't be if you are standing for hours bending over a hot ironing board. Most boards are adjustable and you should be able to lower yours so you are able to sit comfortably and iron, keeping your back as straight as possible.

Incidentally, don't rely on the fact that women in late pregnancy are supposed to feel a 'nesting urge' or 'last burst of energy' to spur you into household chores. If the urge does come at all it is usually pretty short-lived or focused on something quite unnecessary such as washing curtains or scrubbing paintwork.

Arrangements for the Baby

It is not essential that a small baby has a room of her own. If you have the space you are bound to want to make it into a nursery, but if this is not possible you should not feel that your baby is being deprived. All your baby will need in the early weeks of life is a bed of some description (a cot, crib, Moses basket or even a large drawer!) where she will be warm and cozy. In many ways decorating an entire room in what you imagine to be a baby's taste can be a waste of time and money. As soon as your baby becomes a toddler and has likes and dislikes she may not thank you for dreamy pastels and lacy curtains. Although traditionally pastels are said to be relaxing and soothing for a new baby, modern research shows that babies respond earlier to being surrounded by black-and-white objects or simple primary colours.

Most of the basic equipment your baby will need can be bought second-hand if you do not wish or cannot afford to go to the expense of brand-new. Most baby things are used for such a short time before the baby grows out of them that even 'second-hand' items are very nearly new! Essentials are:

- A cot – though at first she will feel more secure in a smaller bed such as a Moses basket or carry-cot (handy for when you take her out). A crib is a luxury as they are expensive and your baby will have grown out of it by six months.
- A changing base: a chest of drawers at the right height with a plastic changing mat is handy as you can keep baby lotion, nappies and so on in the top drawer. It would be wise to keep a supply of glucose tablets there, too, in case you feel hypo in the middle of a nappy change. If you don't have the room for a changing station, a padded plastic mat will suffice.
- A firm, flat mattress (that meets British Kitemark safety standards) with a waterproof cover for whatever kind of bed the baby will sleep in. Never use a pillow as this could cause suffocation.
- If you drive, you will need a rear-facing baby seat with handles that can be secured to the front or back seat of the car.
  Towelling or flannelette fitted sheets.
- A transporter. Prams seem to have been usurped to a large extent by multi-use 'buggies' which can be turned into a carry-cot on wheels, a push-chair/stroller and transportable feeding chair complete with table. New designs come on the market all the time so it's best to shop

around to suit your needs.

- Cotton cellular blankets. These make invaluable top sheets as they allow the baby to breathe if she ends up moving beneath them. A duvet is too bulky for a tiny baby and not recommended until she is strong enough to push it away if it is swamping her.
- Muslin squares to lay under the baby's head to catch any regurgitated milk. Babies can become very attached to their muslins and often end up using them as 'security blankets', so if you are not in favour of 'comforters' then remove muslins if you notice a special attachment forming.
- Nappies – disposable or terry towelling. Consumer research has shown that, taking into account the electricity, etc. used for washing and drying terries there is little difference in the long-term cost compared with disposables. Another option nowadays is a nappy service, which can deliver a weekly supply of nappies, take the soiled ones away and launder them for you (their laundering methods are environmentally sound). They also supply you with outer 'wraps' that have velcro fasteners, thereby doing away with the hassle of pins, plastic pants, etc. Many mothers find this kind of service an environmentally friendly and affordable option, as the weekly fee is the same (if not less) than the price of the better disposables. To find out if there is a nappy service in your area, contact the National Association of Nappy Services (see Useful Addresses).
- If you are going to use disposable nappies then make sure you choose the right size, as tiny babies in huge disposables feel most uncomfortable. If you use terries and are going to clean them yourself you will need at least two dozen good-quality nappies...it's a false economy buying cheap ones as they simply will not last. Don't forget plastic buckets with lids (two) and half a dozen large nappy pins. You may also need good quality plastic pants if using terries and these should be handwashed to minimize disintegration (the velcro wraps used by nappy services can also

be purchased for your own use – see Useful Addresses).
* A baby bath with a stand, although this is not essential...you can use a sink or washing-up bowl until your baby is big enough to feel secure in a normal bath.
* Soft towels, preferably hooded for after the bath.
* A good brand of baby lotion, soap, nappy cream, wet wipes and shampoo (if there's enough hair to wash!). Babies do not need any soap at first, but from around the age of two months a very mild brand can be used.
* A bag that is big enough to hold all nappies, etc. when you go out (plus your diabetes equipment!) – one that unrolls into a waterproof changing mat is particularly good.
* If you are not going to be breastfeeding you will need a sterilizing system and set of six bottles. If you feel uncomfortable or superstitious about having a baby's paraphernalia in the home when, as yet, there is no actual baby around (and a great number of women do feel like this), many department stores will help you to select equipment and keep your order until you notify them that all is well and then they will deliver.

Clothes for your Baby

Try not to be tempted by trendy clothing for tiny babies; you cannot put a minute baby into a denim jacket even if the shop assistant tells you otherwise! Until a baby is at least six months old then there is nothing more practical than stretch suits which can be washed and dried quickly and do not need to be ironed (you will need about half a dozen of these). In the case of clothing, choose pale rather than bright colours as a new-born baby's skin tends to be rather florid and blotchy for the first few weeks of life.

Cotton nighties (two or three) make nappy-changing easier at night, and vests with wide envelope necks and poppers at the bottom will keep your baby warm and help the nappy stay neatly in place.

A close-knit shawl, bonnets, cotton socks or booties, cardigans or jumpers with wide necks are the only other things your baby will need.

You are bound to be given frilly dresses and all kinds of other garments which are quite unsuitable for a new baby, though forward-thinking friends will buy the larger sizes that a fast-growing baby will be able to use later on. Frilly dresses for tiny babies invariably end up as doll's clothes.

Packing Your Bag for the Hospital

Have a small suitcase packed and ready with everything you need for the hospital from week 36 onwards. There is always a chance you could go into labour earlier than expected and in the excitement could very easily forget all sorts of things. You will need some of your diabetes equipment but as you will be using your blood-test kit and insulin until you go it's a good idea to make a list and tape it to the inside of the suitcase lid so you don't leave vital supplies behind.

This list should remind you to take:

- Insulin
- Insulin pen or syringes
- Blood/urine test strips and meter (if you use one)
- Log-book for blood/urine test results
- Glucose tablets

Although the hospital could supply insulins, testing strips, etc. it is far more useful to have everything immediately available. You may find that the nurses take the insulin away and give it back when your injections are due – some hospitals have a safety of medicines policy that stipulates that all personal equipment should be taken.

Keep a suitcase ready with:

- Two or three nightdresses (preferably cotton) with front-openings
- Maternity bras (two or three) with front fastenings
- Lightweight dressing gown
- Slippers or flip-flops
- Several packets of disposable pants (it may be inconvenient to wash out ordinary pants in hospital)
- Super-absorbent sanitary towels; choose the stick-on variety rather than those with loops
- Breast pads and nipple cream
- A washbag with soap, toothpaste and brush, talcum powder, make-up, shampoo and conditioner, flannel or sponge, moisturizer, cotton wool, a mirror and a hand-towel
- Tissues
- Stationery for letter-writing
- A good paperback
- Money for snacks and the telephone (or a phonecard)

Some hospitals supply cotton nighties and nappies for the baby, although with health cuts this is becoming the exception rather than the rule. Find out beforehand exactly what you are (or are not) expected to provide for the baby – they usually supply you with a list. In any case you will need a set of clothes (plus bonnet and shawl) to take the baby home in, but your partner or a friend could always bring this along after the baby is born/when you are ready to take her home.

Decide what clothes you are going to leave hospital in and either add them to your diabetes equipment list for packing or tell whoever will be bringing you home exactly where they will be. Don't be too ambitious and imagine you will get into your pre-pregnancy clothes immediately after the birth; you will only be disappointed, however much weight you appear to have lost. Choose something comfortable and stretchy.

Food and Drink for the Hospital

You will need supplies of sugar-free drinks, biscuits and other suitable snacks to tide you over in hospital. Have a couple of bottles of squash, packets of biscuits, a bag of chocolate mini-bars in case your blood glucose levels are low and anything else you may fancy ready in a plastic bag next to the suitcase. Hospital canteens and food trollies sometimes keep unreliable hours so you can't rely on the hospital to meet your snack-time requirements.

If you have a partner, relative or friend (otherwise known as a 'birth assistant') make sure he or she has another kit consisting of:

- A natural sponge or flannel to keep you cool during labour
- Glucose tablets
- A small cassette/CD player with your favourite tapes (take headphones in case the hospital don't allow music to be played out loud)
- A bottle of still mineral water to sip during labour

Make Arrangements Well Ahead of Time

You must have a plan of action for when you go into labour; things invariably happen at unexpected and often inconvenient times. Have contact numbers for your partner (or birth assistant) at all times – modern technology now means some people even carry bleepers so they can be paged and summoned wherever they happen to be (these can be hired on a weekly basis from British Telecom shops or private advertisers).

Water-tight arrangements must be made for your other children if you have them. Make sure they know well in advance exactly who will be looking after them, picking them up from school (you may need to inform the school) and what the pro-

144

posed plan of action is likely to be. A close relative, friend or nanny/mother's help if you have one is obviously the best choice for this. Whatever happens, your child or children should not feel left out of the preparations and should be made to feel involved and grown up. They will be used to your growing bigger and feeling their new brother or sister move inside you – this is a very important part of the bonding process between siblings. Try to disrupt their routine as little as possible; if they can be looked after in their own home while you are away, so much the better. It's as well to explain in advance to a young child that a new-born baby is not going to be an instant playmate and that, however much he or she is longing to have a new and special instant friend, the new baby will inevitably seem rather boring at first. She will sleep, cry and feed; she will not talk, run around or play computers. If you help your child to understand this before you bring the baby home there will be no disappointment and complaints that the baby does not live up to expectations.

Going into Labour

As time edges towards the date that your baby is due to be born you are bound to be apprehensive. In some cases women are taken into hospital and induced at 38 weeks (see Chapter 11) if there appear to be any risks involved in letting the pregnancy go to full term. But with more and more understanding and good management of diabetes in pregnancy this is becoming far less likely than in the past. If this is your first pregnancy you may wonder how labour is going to begin; indeed, whether you will actually recognize the signs that it has started! If you have been attending antenatal classes then you will have learned the various signs that are recognizable as those of early labour. Some women's labour starts slowly, with contractions building up over a period of time; others find that their waters (the amniotic fluid from the womb) break in a sudden gush and they must go into hospital straight away. Hopefully you will be prepared (suitcase packed, diabetes equipment ready, other children organized and birth assistant contactable) for any eventuality. Whatever happens you will feel excited and, hopefully, confident. There may be signs during the week or so before labour starts that things are moving towards delivery day:

- Passing water frequently as the baby's head puts pressure on the bladder (though you should check that high blood glucose levels are not the reason for this).
- Braxton Hicks contractions (see Chapter 5) become more frequent and you may think they are actual contractions of labour. If in doubt, call your antenatal clinic who will be able to tell from your description whether labour is beginning. In fact, Braxton Hicks contractions cause only slight discomfort and are less frequent than true labour pains.
- You may feel a euphoric burst of energy which spurs you on to spring-cleaning.
- Slight weight loss is often a sign that something is about to happen.
- You may notice an increase in vaginal secretions, rather like a discharge, a few days before labour starts.

Recognizing Labour When it Begins

There are three classic and very recognizable symptoms of the beginning of labour which, once you experience them, cannot be mistaken: rupture of the membranes, a 'show', and powerful contractions.

Rupture of the Membranes (Breaking of the Waters)
This is painless and feels like a popping sensation, apparently in the anus. If the baby's head has not yet engaged you may

lose a larger quantity of fluid from the vagina than if it is low down in the pelvis. In either event it will probably be quite a noticeable amount (even a steady trickle is recognizable). Although it is unlikely that you will start contractions straight away (it could be anything up to 12 hours), you should phone the hospital immediately for instructions as you will almost certainly be asked to go in once the waters have broken. If your insulin injection and meal are due, you will probably be told to carry on as normal. You may feel too excited to eat but you must take your insulin and 'cover' it with enough carbohydrates.

I actually felt quite relaxed about the whole thing and wanted to take my time. But the hospital insisted I go right in and told me that I would be given intravenous insulin and glucose so not to bother with breakfast, which was still two hours away when my waters broke. I felt very hassled, although once I was there and all wired up I relaxed again.

The 'Show'

A 'show' is a small amount of pinkish blood mixed with mucus. This is in fact the dislodged 'plug' (a solid lump of clear, sticky mucus) from the cervix, which occurs before the onset of labour or in its first stages. This is quite normal and, again, you should inform the hospital while carrying on with your diabetes routine. Some women experience a 'show' a day or two before they actually go into labour.

Contractions

These may feel like crampy period pains or a low, nagging backache with a tightening of the abdomen. They may even feel like the sharp discomfort you experience with an attack of diarrhoea. If you feel a wave of discomfort across your stomach which reaches a peak and then fades away, put your hand on your stomach and you will feel a hardening and then relaxing of the muscle which controls the uterus.

It's easier said than done, perhaps, but the more relaxed you feel in yourself, the less painful these contractions will be. Take note of the time between each contraction and phone the hospital for advice. They may tell you to sit tight and keep timing your contractions until they are coming frequently and lasting, in the early stages of labour, between 30 and 60 seconds from the start of one contraction to the beginning of the next. As you have diabetes, you may be told to come in immediately so the situation can be assessed at the hospital.

I have to admit that I panicked. The midwife was quite happy for me to stay at home until my contractions were established and regular and told me to have my insulin and lunch. I couldn't cope with having to think about what to eat and timing contractions so I called them back and said please could I go in right then...

If there has been any worry about the position of the baby and any mention of a Caesarean section (see Chapter 11) you will certainly need to go straight to hospital and, in this case, will be given special instructions as to whether to inject/eat, etc. A first baby usually causes the longest labour (around 12–14 hours) and the lighter the contractions, the longer labour is likely to be. Slow, strong contractions tend to point towards a quick birth. Contractions do not always follow a pattern; you may have a strong one followed by a weaker one and you may even find that there is little gap between them so they keep on coming one after the other, incessantly. Breathing techniques that you have learned at antenatal classes (or those in Chapter 8) and any other methods you can use to relax will be a great help at this time.

However labour begins – whether spontaneously or induced – you will suddenly feel full of energy however tired you may have felt beforehand. Adrenalin will be pumping round your body (blood glucose levels may well go up again). After all those weeks and months of waiting, your baby is now ready to be born.

Chapter 11

WHEN THE BIG DAY ARRIVES

What to Expect in Hospital

Once you arrive at the hospital you will be admitted and shown to your bed. A midwife will examine you and she can determine how far labour has actually advanced. She will also check your pulse, temperature and blood pressure. You will probably be asked to check your own blood glucose levels at certain times and to keep a record of these in the form of a chart. If for some reason (say, if contractions are very close together) you can't manage this yourself, you will be given help. By feeling your abdomen the midwife will be able to establish the position of the baby and she may also carry out an internal examination. Depending on the policy of the hospital, you may be given an enema or suppository so you can empty your bowels and your pubic hair may be shaved (although these practices are less and less common these days).

Remember that any form of stress or excitement can raise your blood glucose levels, so try and do some deep breathing exercises to calm yourself down! In any event, your blood glucose levels will be monitored, so you will be able to tell how they are reacting to the excitement.

If you have been on insulin during your pregnancy you will be put on an insulin infusion pump which involves a needle being inserted into your arm, with a tube attached to it. The tube is connected to an insulin pump and a bag of dextrose (a form of sugar). Depending on your blood glucose levels, the midwife will either give you more insulin or more dextrose directly into your bloodstream, allowing your diabetes to be carefully controlled throughout labour. It is also likely a foetal monitor will be attached to your stomach (or sometimes to the baby's head) to record his heart rate and the pressure of your contractions. If the baby becomes distressed during labour, his heart rate will alter and the midwife will be able to see what's happening on the monitor and speed up labour if necessary.

Unfortunately, all this paraphernalia will restrict your movements but you must remember they are important for the health and well-being of you and your baby.

I have to say it wasn't the kind of birth one would fantasize about. Before I became diabetic five years earlier I used to have this vision of myself walking around freely, Le Boyer style, and squatting to have a baby. In the event, I was trussed up like a chicken! But I had no objections – I knew what had to happen and as my baby was seen to be in distress resulting in a forceps delivery I was very relieved that I was given the high-tech birth! The thing was, I felt completely confident even when his heart rate and my blood glucose levels went wild.

Once labour is under way and your baby is about to come into the world, you will be moved to a delivery room. The midwife will be with you and there may also be a paediatrician (who specializes in looking after babies and children). Your birth partner will be encouraged to help while you are in labour by reminding you of your breathing exercises, rubbing your back to help you to get you through any pain, and simply being there for you.

How your diabetes reacts to labour is, of course, very individual. However, you will be monitored so carefully that any event can be rectified immediately by adjusting the dextrose (or insulin) drips.

Eating is definitely out (you probably won't feel hungry anyway!) One reason for this is that some women find food makes them sick during labour, but the most important reason is that if you need a Caesarean section with a general anaesthetic there is a real risk of vomiting anything you might have eaten once you are under anaesthetic. You may well feel thirsty and sips of water are generally fine.

Pain Relief

There are various forms of pain relief available in labour; these will have been explained to you at antenatal classes. Being educated and informed about what to expect in labour will go a long way towards allaying any fears you may have – that's why attending antenatal classes is such a good idea (see Chapter 3).

The choice of which kind of pain relief to opt for is entirely yours – you may well feel you want to 'go it alone' and have a so-called 'natural' birth using only the breathing and relaxation techniques you have been taught. Don't let anyone impose his or her beliefs on you regarding pain relief, and never feel guilty for any decision you eventually make.

Not all women require drugs during labour, particularly if they have had children before. Naturally, first-time mothers may feel more anxious especially if they have heard lurid tales from others which may well have become exaggerated with the passage of time. It's a good idea to keep an open mind and not dismiss out of hand any notion that you might change your mind at the last minute. Incidentally, there is no evidence that pain-relieving drugs have any effect on glucose levels during labour.

I had been convinced at my antenatal classes that I would have a completely natural birth using only my relaxation techniques to get me through. Once in labour I begged for an epidural and luckily the anaesthetist could be contacted in time. There was no messing about for my second delivery – I booked the epidural weeks ahead!

Your partner or birth assistant and the hospital staff should also play an important role in reassuring you. It's a good idea if you and your partner or friend practise and perfect the breathing exercises you will learn in antenatal classes before the big day arrives so you can avoid any panic! Remember that the midwife will be at the birth to guide you whether you have a partner with you or not, so there will be no need to feel alone.

Most drugs given during labour cross the placental barrier and, to some extent, have the same effect on the baby as they do on the mother. During early labour only, a sedative may be given which allows the woman to relax and perhaps get some sleep so she can build up her strength. This, however, would not be a painkiller.

The Options

Pethidine

This is the most commonly used analgesic (painkiller) used in labour. It is given by injection once labour has been established. It starts to work about 15 minutes after it has been given and is effective up to about four hours. Not only does it relieve pain but it can also induce a feeling of well-being and high spirits. Not all women find they are completely free of pain but the pethidine helps relaxation which allows labour to progress. The side-effects are sometimes nausea, vomiting and drowsiness which may prevent you from pushing when you have to. As far as the baby is concerned, pethidine should not be given within an hour of delivery as it can make him drowsy and slow to breathe (although this can be rectified if it should happen). Some women have found that pethidine brings on feelings of confusion rather than euphoria, but again it is very individual and unfortunately there is no way of knowing beforehand how this drug will affect you.

When I had pethidine during labour with my first baby, I found the experience quite distressing. I felt disorientated and not in control. Other women I've talked to didn't find it so bad, so maybe mine was just an unusual reaction – I'd already been up for about 20 hours before I was given it, so maybe that was part of the problem!

Gas and Air

This is a combination of the gas nitrous oxide and oxygen which is stored in a cylinder. Attached to this is a face mask or a mouth-piece. Your aim is to inhale the gas and air when you feel a contraction coming so the effect of the gas works just when the contraction is at its most painful. *You* are in control of the mask and so you can use it as required. This can take some practice to get right and although this form of analgesia does not block the pain completely, it is fairly effective. Gas and air is often used in conjunction with pethidine.

There are no side-effects of gas and air for you or your baby. However, gas and air may make you feel nauseous and sleepy; the mask can also make some women feel claustrophobic and disorientated, which can be a drawback in the second stage of labour when you need to really concentrate on your contractions and push.

Epidural

An epidural block involves inserting a needle into the spinal canal and injecting a local anaesthetic, thereby numbing the spinal nerves which carry the sensation of pain. Along with the needle a very fine tube (or catheter) is inserted. When the needle is removed one end of the tube remains in the spinal canal; the other end is strapped to your back so that anaesthetic can be topped up through the tube as you need it. Pain relief lasts between two and four hours; the more anaesthetic used, the greater the pain relief. In the majority of cases, epidurals provide complete pain relief and an effective form of relaxation to help labour progress smoothly, plus there are no side-effects for the baby.

You, however, may find it difficult to move and your legs will certainly feel heavy. Some women feel rather sick and dizzy with an epidural as it can lower the blood pressure considerably. As you can no longer feel your contractions, the midwife or obstetrician will have to tell you when to push. An epidural must always and *only* be given by an anaesthetist. As some hospitals don't have an anaesthetist on call 24 hours a day, you may need to book one in advance so that when you go into labour the anaesthetist will be contacted. The disadvantage to this is that you may have wanted to manage without an epidural and not booked an anaesthetist. It could then be touch and go as to whether an anaesthetist can get to you – in some cases you may not be able to get one at all.

An epidural can also be used instead of a general anaesthetic. A great bonus is that in a Caesarean section this allows you to be awake during the delivery yet feel no pain. Your partner or helper can also be with you whereas he or she would not be allowed to be present at an operation when a general anaesthetic is given.

A spinal block is similar to an epidural except that only one injection of anaesthetic can be given during labour. The effect lasts about two hours. This can also be used for Caesareans (instead of a general anaesthetic), or if a forceps delivery is required. In the past, spinal blocks usually caused severe headaches; today a change in the anaesthesia used has minimized this problem.

Whatever you decide, it is your personal choice. You are entitled to change your mind once labour has started so, as we advised earlier, try to keep an open mind and don't let anyone force a decision on you. This is *your* baby and the choice of pain relief is yours.

Stages of Labour

No one understands exactly what actually causes labour to begin, but it is generally assumed to be due to a sudden release of hormones from the placenta.

The process of labour is divided into three stages.

First Stage

This is from the very beginning of labour until the cervix – or neck of the womb – is fully dilated and becomes wide enough to allow the baby's head to pass through. During this first stage the uterus, which is an incredibly strong muscle, contracts causing the cervix to open up to about 10 cm/4 in. Your midwife will check regularly to see how far the cervix has dilated. During this early stage the midwife may not be able to be with you all the time – but if for any reason you feel worried, use the call system to attract her attention. If you suddenly feel the urge to push – which is a sensation rather like opening the bowels – you must let the midwife know immediately.

The length of the first stage of labour varies from woman to woman. At the beginning things may progress very slowly and it's easy to imagine nothing is happening. If this is your first baby, this first stage is likely to last between 0 and 12 hours. For subsequent babies the first stage, on average, lasts about 6 hours. Sometimes a drip or pessaries containing hormones are given to help speed things up if they are going particularly slowly.

Second Stage

This stage is from full dilation of the cervix to the complete delivery of the baby.

Once the cervix is fully dilated the baby's head is able to pass into the vagina and this is the time you may feel like you want to push. If you have been given an epidural you may not feel this sensation at all, but with regular checks the midwife will be able to tell how imminent the birth actually is. With each contraction, take a few deep breaths and push down as if you were on the toilet – the vagina will stretch to accommodate the baby's head. This stage of labour is where the really hard work comes in, but whoever is in the room with you will certainly do their best to encourage you!

The midwife should explain what is happening every step of the way, but if there's anything you want to ask, don't be afraid to speak up. The second stage of labour lasts about 1 to 2 hours depending on whether this is your first baby or not. When the midwife can see the top of the baby's head at the entrance to the vagina (the 'crowning'), she will tell you to pause and stop pushing. You will then be urged to push *very* gently or 'pant' (something you will have been taught at antenatal classes) so that the head can come out slowly. This restraining action is to prevent the area between your vagina and your back passage (the perineum) from tearing; by delivering the head slowly there is less chance of this happening. If the perineum does not stretch enough, you may be given an episiotomy – a local anaesthetic is administered and the skin of the perineum is cut. After delivery is complete this cut will be stitched up. If the perineum should get torn this will also be stitched up after delivery. Neither a tear nor an episiotomy causes any lasting problems with the perineum – many women who have had an episiotomy with their first baby find that for later births the perineum stretches perfectly well on its own.

Once the baby has crowned and the head is delivered, the rest of the birth is easier. One last push is usually enough to bring the baby fully into the world! The baby will probably be laid in your arms so you can be close to each other straight away. On first impressions new babies can often look alarming; they are sometimes blue, covered with a white cheesy-looking substance (called vernix) and rather slippery with streaks of blood (yours) all over. Any hair they may have will be stuck greasily to the head. New-born babies are *not* the round, pink pretty little beings you see on adverts. Your baby could well look a bit squashed – even bruised if you have had a forceps delivery – but remember, he has had a hard journey. His nose, throat and mouth may need to be cleared to enable him to take his first breath and he may need some oxygen to help get his breathing going. If you do have to be separated from your baby, it will be for as short a time as possible.

The minute the baby starts breathing normally, his colour will be pink and natural. Unless he has been taken away to be given help for his breathing, you will still be joined by the umbilical cord. This must now be clamped and cut; once this has been done your baby will be an entirely separate person, functioning independently.

If you are going to breastfeed, let your baby suckle as soon as possible. The midwife will encourage this and will help you latch the baby onto your breast. It's amazing that babies begin to suckle even when they have just been born; this will help with feeding later on. It also causes the uterus to contract and begin to go back to its normal size.

You will no doubt be filled with awe and wonder at this new life. You may feel total love for your new baby from the minute he is born, yet not every woman feels this pleasure immediately. This is something that you must try not to worry about. Everyone reacts differently and sometimes circumstances dictate that a loving bond is not always spontaneous

After a long labour and Chloe being taken to special care, I felt exhausted and, frankly, not much of a new mum. I wanted to see Chloe but when I did I couldn't relate to her at all. I felt very

strange for the first few days – it was only when we left the hospi-
tal that the love for this tiny creature really enveloped me.

Third Stage

This final stage of labour is when the placenta comes away
from the wall of the uterus and is pushed out by the mother or
removed by the midwife. The delivery of the placenta lasts
from about three to five minutes. The midwife will probably
give you an injection, just after the baby has been born to help
the uterus contract, and thus expel the placenta.

If you have needed an episiotomy or the perineum has been
torn, you will have some stitches. Last but not least, the midwife or your birth partner will help you wash and freshen up,
ready to be taken back to the hospital ward and your bed.

Complications Which May Arise

Induction

This means bringing on labour artificially and there are a
number of reasons for doing this – if the baby is overdue, large
for dates or there is some risk to either mother or baby (for
example, if the mother has high blood pressure). In the past,
women with diabetes were induced at 38 weeks routinely, just
in case the baby became too big. But modern thinking now
means that providing there are no problems and mother and
baby are well monitored then the pregnancy can usually go
full term. The decision will be the obstetrician's.

Andry was induced for both her babies at 38 weeks:

My blood glucose levels were very well controlled throughout my pregnancies and I had regular scans which showed all was well. For these reasons I wanted to go into labour naturally but the doctor insisted the babies should be born as soon as possible. I felt that my doctors had no confidence in dealing with diabetic pregnancies and hope that this has changed with progress.

Inducing labour is done either by breaking the waters (artificial rupture of the membranes) or by inserting a pessary containing hormones into the vagina or a hormone drip into the arm. After being induced, labour can proceed as normal. Other implications of having a hormonal drip are that your blood pressure will be checked regularly and that the contractions may be more intense than usual, a situation that will normally be dealt with by epidural block.

Forceps Delivery

Forceps are used to aid the birth of the baby if, for example, contractions are not strong enough to push the baby out, the foetal monitor shows that the baby is distressed, or the midwife becomes aware of other signs that all is not progressing as it might. It is rare that the mother becomes distressed, but too much exertion while bearing down to push can cause this. There may be other medical reasons which the doctor feels are important enough to warrant using forceps.

Forceps are made to fit over the baby's head and will not do any harm. You may notice afterwards some red marks on the baby's head where the forceps have been, but these disappear within a few hours of the birth.

Vacuum or Ventouse Extraction

This can be used as an alternative to forceps. A small metal cup is passed into the vagina and attached to the baby's head by suction. The gentle suction allows the baby to be pulled out, while you push. When he is born the baby will have a swelling on his head where the cup has been, but this soon disappears.

Caesarean Section

There are many reasons for a Caesarean section. About 25–30 per cent of diabetic deliveries are by Caesarean, and it is the obstetrician who will decide whether or not to perform this operation to deliver the baby through the wall of the abdomen. Caesareans are either 'elective' (planned) or 'emergency' (the decision is only made during labour). An elective Caesarean may be performed because the baby's position is too awkward for a vaginal delivery. Sometimes the mother's pelvis is considered too small to accommodate a normal delivery. Whatever the reason, an elective Caesarean will be performed if vaginal delivery is considered too much of a risk to either mother or baby. These circumstances actually apply whether you have diabetes or not. If you have been told you will need a Caesarean you will go into hospital at around 38 to 39 weeks, so there is very little risk you will go into labour spontaneously before your baby is delivered by Caesarean.

An emergency Caesarean may be necessary when a normal delivery is not progressing as it should. For example, if the baby is in distress and needs to be born quickly.

A Caesarean can either be performed under general anaesthetic, in which case you will be unconscious, or with an epidural to allow you to remain awake and 'participate' in the birth. If you remain awake, a screen will be placed across you so you will not actually be able to see the operation happening – although it is worth mentioning that even the sound of a

Caesarean can sometimes cause a woman a certain amount of distress. Many hospitals allow the birthing partner to be in the operating theatre with the mother if she is not having a general anaesthetic – and of course the great advantage of having an epidural and staying awake during the operation is that you are able to see your baby as soon as it is born.

To perform a Caesarean section, the obstetrician makes an incision (usually horizontal) below the 'bikini line'. The resulting scar will eventually be covered over by pubic hair. The time it takes from the first incision to the baby being born is around 10 minutes and the procedure after the baby is lifted from the abdomen is virtually the same as with a vaginal delivery (unless of course you have had a general anaesthetic, in which case you will not see the baby until you have come round). The whole operation including sewing up the incision takes about 45 minutes to an hour. You will be given an injection for any pain and you are bound to find your Caesarean scar rather uncomfortable for a while. Certainly, getting up and about is not as easy as it is after a vaginal delivery. Once the stitches or clips have been removed (between the fifth and seventh day) you will probably be able to go home, providing your diabetes is reasonably well controlled.

A Caesarean may seem a very 'unnatural' sort of birth but most women who have had them report that once they have their baby the elation they feel minimizes the 'surgical' nature of the birth.

After the Delivery

Whether you have a vaginal delivery or a Caesarean your baby will be examined by the midwife or obstetrician to make sure that he is fit and healthy. A healthy baby will breathe soon after delivery and his lungs will expand when he cries. In fact, a baby's first cry symbolizes his physical transformation to the outside world. As soon as the baby is born, the midwife or obstetrician will examine the baby to determine the 'Apgar' score. This shows a rating which takes into account factors such as the baby's muscle tone, strength, heart rate, colour and other factors. The Apgar score is repeated at 2, 5 and 10 minutes after the birth, which tells the medical team if the baby needs help in any of the relevant areas.

Your baby will also be examined again – usually by the midwife – for congenital abnormalities. If anything is discovered, the paediatrician will also examine the baby. Once these routine checks have shown all is well, you will go to the postnatal ward where you will be given help in looking after your new baby. You may not even be sure how to change a nappy if this is your first child. But don't worry: however strange it seems you will gain confidence very quickly.

Special Care

As we discussed at the beginning of this book, some babies born to mothers who have diabetes are large and sometimes 'flaccid' or floppy. If this is the case then you can still have the baby beside you but he will be carefully observed by the staff. Every baby born to a mother with diabetes will have a blood glucose test after delivery via a prick on the heel of the baby's foot to make sure he is not hypoglycaemic (which can happen because of the baby's delayed response in adapting to a glucose-free environment while he is still producing insulin on his own). If the baby is hypo, he will still go with you to the ward but he will need to be fed frequently to raise his blood glucose levels. If your baby is not feeding well and his blood glucose levels are low he will need to be transferred to the special care baby unit and will be given dextrose through a drip. This will only be for a short time, until his pancreas adapts and he produces the right amount of insulin to match the amount of milk he takes.

Naturally, having your baby taken to the special care unit is a worrying experience. But remember that these units are run by an experienced team of midwives who are trained to look after babies with special needs. Knowing what is going on and making sure you have enough information which you understand will help alleviate some of the stress. When the doctor explains what is happening, try to have your partner or someone close to you with you so you do not misinterpret what has been said or miss any important points. Make sure you ask questions – don't leave any stone unturned in your understanding of the problem.

Special care units can look daunting: there is a lot of unfamiliar high-tech equipment and your baby may be attached to drips and monitors. You will certainly be encouraged to visit your baby and, if possible, hold and feed him. If you want to breastfeed but your baby is unable to manage this at first you can express your milk (your midwife will explain how to do this) and this can then be given to your baby by bottle.

When All Is Not Well

One should not ignore the fact that some pregnancies result in the baby being born handicapped. Some parents only discover their baby has a handicap weeks or months after the birth. If this unfortunate situation should occur you should not assume that it has something to do with your having diabetes, as this may well not be the case at all. The important thing is that you have all the help and support you can get and you should ask your midwife, paediatrician and health visitor for information.

It is a distressing fact that sometimes a pregnancy ends in

stillbirth or the death of a baby soon after birth. Why this happens is often unknown; thankfully it only happens in a very small number of cases. A post-mortem would have to be carried out to try and determine the cause, but frequently the questions are left unanswered. Again, try not to imagine that diabetes is the cause, though naturally you will want to try and find out why this has happened. Talk to the midwife, health visitor and doctors; they may not have all the answers but they are there to help you. We have listed the addresses of a number offering support networks for bereaved parents.

Your Diabetes After the Birth

Once delivery is complete and you are eating and drinking again the insulin pump will be turned off and your blood glucose levels should return to normal. If you have had a Caesarean you will remain on a drip until you are able to tolerate fluids and food. Once the drip is removed you may well find that your insulin requirements are less than those you needed before you were pregnant. If you had previously been taking tablets for your diabetes and were put onto insulin for the pregnancy, you may remain on these injections for a few more days, until your blood glucose levels settle down. If you are breastfeeding you will need to remain on insulin, as some tablets used for the treatment of diabetes can be passed through breastmilk and thus cause your baby to become hypo.

The first few days of motherhood can be difficult and, particularly if this is your first baby, you might feel totally bewildered. The midwives will do all they can to help you in the beginning and answer any questions, however trivial you think they may sound. If you feel uncomfortable after having stitches, sitting on a rubber ring might help. Some hospitals recommend ice packs and salt baths to ease the discomfort. Drink plenty of water and make sure your diet is high in fibre to prevent becoming constipated, as this can also be most uncomfortable.

For anything up to six weeks after the birth you will have some vaginal bleeding (whichever kind of delivery you may have had). This is known as 'lochia' and is a discharge of blood and mucus from the uterus. You may notice some clots at the beginning; the flow will become brownish and pale before it stops. Do not use tampons for a few weeks after the birth as there is a risk of infection. Your periods may start as soon as a month after delivery or much later if you are breast-feeding.

Your stay in hospital will last for at least 48 hours after the birth (longer stays depend on the hospital's policy, whether you have had a Caesarean, how your blood glucose levels are settling down, etc.). On leaving, the midwife will examine you and the paediatrician will examine the baby. You will be given a date for your postnatal check-up around six to eight weeks after the birth. Check that the hospital will inform your diabetes team that you have left. They will also tell the community midwife that you have gone home, as she will be visiting you at home for the first 10 days after the birth.

Chapter 12

GETTING BACK TO NORMAL

Going Home

Leaving hospital with your new-born baby is bound to make you feel both excited and nervous at the same time. This is it: you are now going to have to make your own decisions concerning your baby without a midwife standing by to help, although things probably won't seem so strange if this is not your first child. The community midwife will come and visit you for 10 days after the birth (which includes the time you spent in hospital). She will let the health visitor know when her visits have finished, as then your health visitor takes over to help with any problems in looking after the baby (and yourself).

You may also be visited by your diabetes specialist nurse; if she is unable to visit and you have problems with your blood glucose control, make sure you contact her and she will help you sort things out as soon as possible.

In Chapter 11 we talked about blood glucose levels returning to pre-pregnancy levels after delivery – insulin requirements may drop dramatically, even more than you might expect if you are breastfeeding (see later in this chapter). Many women who have insulin-dependent diabetes find themselves a bit muddled, having become used to such high doses.

166

I had got used to 30 units injected before each meal – over 100 units a day – while I was pregnant. My pre-pregnancy dose had been 30 units a day and I kept finding myself injecting too much and then I'd have to stuff my face with carbohydrates so I wouldn't hypo.

Pinning a chart to your kitchen wall with insulin requirements clearly stated will help (see page 170), as will keeping your blood-testing record book with your injection equipment, always having a note of the relevant dose for each meal or time of day, and checking before you inject – mistakes are easy to make in the haze of new motherhood!

Baby Blues

It's very common to feel down in the dumps and tearful about three or four days following the birth. This is known as 'baby' or 'postpartum' blues and coincides with the beginning of the milk flow – for the first three or so days your breasts will be producing mostly colostrum (see below) until your milk comes in. Your hormones have been at high levels throughout your pregnancy and have now fallen back to normal – it's like a withdrawal of euphoria and may cause you to feel moody and miserable. Try to talk about your feelings – especially to your partner who may be thoroughly confused that after giving birth to a beautiful, healthy baby you are now weepy and depressed. If your feelings won't lighten up and you can't shake anxieties off, please don't hesitate to speak to your GP or health visitor.

You certainly need to look after yourself as well as looking after your baby. Hopefully you will have stocked up on your diabetes supplies – have everything to hand, as your baby will seem to take up all of your thoughts and time. Get your priorities right. If you don't have any help at home, forget the housework for a while or at least keep it to an absolute minimum. Make meals simple so you do not have to spend your precious spare time slaving over a hot stove. However, don't forget about eating well as you need a good, healthy diet to keep you going. Having diabetes means you must eat, which is only right for any new mother. A healthy diet is also very important if you are breastfeeding, as you will be using up more energy (see page 171).

Getting Enough Rest

Childbirth is an exhausting enough experience, yet some women find the early days at home with a new baby (the first, particularly) far more overwhelming than the actual delivery. One of the physical reasons for the overpowering exhaustion you may feel afterwards is that the volume of blood circulating in your body has been cut by around 30 per cent after delivery and for a while there is not sufficient blood to reach the muscles and make them perform sufficiently. That's why even the smallest tasks often take on the perspective of climbing a mountain! On top of that, you have to get up at night to feed the baby, run a home and, perhaps, look after other children as well as this unpredictable and demanding new addition to your life. With diabetes to cope with on top of everything else it would be pretty surprising if you did not feel overwhelmed and worn out. It may be a tall order, but making sure you get as much rest and sleep as possible in the first days is essential. At least in hospital you don't have to worry about meals and shopping. You also have other new mums around to chat to and share experiences with...no wonder so many new mothers feel scared stiff when the time comes to go home. Many find that they are still in their dressing gowns well into the afternoon!

I had been out of hospital just a couple of days and my 3-year-old son wanted to go to MacDonalds. I thought this would do us both good and give us a chance to be on our own together. I struggled out of my dressing gown, left the new baby with my husband and off we went. First, I couldn't seem to remember where MacDonalds was, secondly I forgot my insulin but worst of all I literally froze while crossing the main road. Poor Peter was crying and trying to drag me across...we had stopped on a traffic island and I couldn't move. At first I thought I was having a hypo but once someone helped us across I recovered and realized it was complete disorientation. In those few days after having the baby I seemed to have forgotten how to do the simplest things. My brain seemed to be scrambled through lack of sleep.

If you can, aim to sleep whenever the baby sleeps. This may be quite possible to achieve if you have some back-up help to look after other children (partner, friend, relation, hired help). If you are on your own with the baby try and organize your own meals to fit round her feeds. In case your baby sleeps through her feed, make sure you set an alarm clock so you don't become hypo because you have also slept through a meal or snack-time. Always have snacks and glucose tablets by your side. You might have been an extremely well-organized person before the birth, but Sandra's description of 'scrambled brain' rings true with many new mothers and you *must* look after your diabetes. Draw up a chart of your injection times, insulin doses, meal and snack-times. Make it large and clear, then pin it to the wall in the kitchen so you and others can see what you are supposed to be doing and when (see illustration below). Friends and relatives will be longing to see the new baby and the phone is bound to ring constantly with would-be visitors. Without appearing anti-social, try to discourage this if you feel exhausted or at least ask them to help out by doing some shopping for you on the way, making their own cups of tea while they visit, etc. The most important thing is to *put yourself and your new baby first* during these early days. Like so many other women you could find motherhood a badly-lit tunnel...finding your way through it may be difficult but you'll learn as you go along and suddenly see the light at the end.

INSULIN! DON'T FORGET IT!

Pre - Breakfast	6 units soluble
Pre - Lunch	6 units soluble
Pre - Dinner	8 units soluble
Before Bed	15 units isophane

Sample wall chart of injection times and doses

Breastfeeding

During your pregnancy and for a few days after the birth your breasts produce a liquid called colostrum. This often looks yellow and is thicker than breastmilk. Colostrum provides proteins and antibodies and is a good source of nourishment for a new baby. When the actual milk comes in (on about day three) your breasts will become large and feel unbelievably heavy. Make sure you wear a good nursing bra which gives enough support. You will also need to put breast pads into your bra to absorb any leaking milk, though this will settle down. You may find breastfeeding difficult in the beginning, but try to persevere as breastmilk is the best food for babies. There are many other advantages to breastfeeding as well.

- Breastmilk is natural and provides the right nutrients for the baby. It is easily digested as it varies in strength at different times of the day to meet the baby's needs.
- The protein which breastmilk contains builds up the baby's muscles and the fat is used for energy and warmth. Breastfed babies tend not to become fat and flabby.
- Breastmilk contains antibodies which help prevent allergies such as asthma and eczema.
- Breastmilk is clean and readily available. It is always the right temperature and it's free!
- Breastfeeding helps the uterus to contract, which is a help in getting your figure back. You actually use some of the extra fat acquired in pregnancy to make milk.
- Some studies suggest feeding the baby yourself reduces the risk of breast cancer later in life.
- Breastfeeding provides a very special closeness between you and your baby.

Each time you feed your baby, make sure you have eaten some form of carbohydrate and always keep some near you. Breastfeeding uses 600–900 calories a day so you will need to keep up your carbohydrate intake to prevent yourself becoming hypo. As feeding becomes established your baby will take more milk so you will need more carbohydrates. You may also find you need to reduce your insulin – some women find their requirements drop by up to 25 per cent.

Breastfeeding can make you thirsty, so a glass of milk or unsweetened orange juice will serve a dual purpose if you would rather not eat; carbohydrate in the form of drinks is quick and easy, particularly when you have to get up for night feeds. However, if you are organized (and hungry!) you may prefer to make a sandwich and leave it in the fridge until you need it during the night. On average, you will need around 50 g/1.5 oz extra carbohydrate every day.

Babies vary in their feeding patterns: some are hungry every 1–1½ hours, some just every 4 hours. It shouldn't be too long before your baby settles into a routine and the time between feeds will become longer. Breastfeeding means you cannot have any way of knowing how much milk your baby is getting and, in turn, how much carbohydrate you require. Checking your blood glucose levels before and after each feed will provide the answer to this problem, although it's not advisable to keep your blood glucose levels as tightly controlled as during your pregnancy – you may run the risk of hypos, which you certainly don't want right now!

When it's time to feed your baby, make sure you are both relaxed and comfortable. If you have had a Caesarean you may find lying on your side easier to start with. Putting a pillow under the baby if you sit up to feed her can also make breastfeeding more comfortable for you. Positioning your baby correctly on the breast is very important. Make sure the baby does not take just the nipple into her mouth but as much of the areola (the dark area around the nipple) as possible. If she sucks only on the nipple, it may become cracked and sore. The milk ducts lie just under the areola so the sensation of the baby's mouth moving on the areola stimulates the milk up through the nipple. When you first start to breastfeed, the midwife will help you to latch your baby onto the breast; once she is feeding correctly you will notice her mouth is wide open and her lower lip curled back below the base of the nipple. Breastfeeding does not always come naturally, so make use of advisory services (some hospitals have breastfeeding counsellors, so does the National Childbirth Trust) and, of course, your midwife and health visitor.

Mastitis

This is a localized infection of the breast which is usually preceded by a cracked nipple. A cracked nipple will feel very sore and it may hurt so much that you cannot bear to let the baby feed properly. If this should happen you need to rest the nipple and express your milk by hand or pump. You will probably have a temperature and notice reddening of the skin over the infected part of the breast. As an infection usually causes blood glucose levels to rise, make sure you do frequent blood tests and increase your insulin as necessary. Your doctor will probably prescribe antibiotics; as the infection clears up your blood glucose levels will come down, so don't forget to decrease your insulin accordingly.

Bottle Feeding

If for one reason or another – which may well be personal choice – you decide to bottle feed, there is one big advantage: someone else can feed the baby for you, giving you precious time to yourself. The routine of sterilizing and making up bottles does seem time-consuming at first but once you get used to it, there's no problem. You will need as many as six bottles and teats so there are always some ready and sterilized when you need to make up feeds. Your midwife or health visitor will explain the various methods available for sterilizing. It is important to clean and sterilize all bottles and equipment thoroughly to prevent the risk of your baby picking up germs and becoming ill.

Baby milk formula is cow's milk which has been specially treated; there are a number of different brands, most of which come in powder form. There are no antibodies in cow's milk and some babies do develop an allergy to it. If this happens speak to your health visitor; she may suggest you try soya milk.

Bottle feeding does not mean you can't become as close as when you breastfeed. Hold the baby in a way that ensures you are looking into each others' eyes and cuddle her closely to you. *Never* leave her alone with a bottle propped up against a cushion or cot, as this could cause her to choke.

Cot Death

This is also known as Sudden Infant Death Syndrome (SIDS), the cause of which is unknown. Cot Death happens when the baby is asleep, most commonly between the ages of one and five months. Fortunately, it is a comparatively rare event. New evidence has suggested that there are precautions you can take to reduce the risk.

It seems that cot death occurs more frequently in babies who are put to sleep on their tummies. They should be put to sleep either on their backs or on their side with their lower arm forward to stop them rolling forwards. Never put a rolled blanket or sheet behind their back as this may also push them forward. Make sure everyone who looks after your baby knows what position to put her when she goes down to sleep.

Make sure your baby is not too warm – the room temperature should be just comfortable (the recommended temperature is 21°C/70°F until the baby is 1 month old and 16°C/60°F afterwards; make sure she is cool in summer with very light, if any, covering). Never use a duvet or baby nest which can cover a baby's head and suffocate her – lightweight blankets, especially cellular ones, are easy to layer or remove if necessary. Some babies do have medical problems which mean they have to sleep on their tummies; if this is the case and you are worried, talk to your doctor, midwife or health visitor. Once your baby is able to roll over by herself she is safe to sleep whichever way she prefers. Incidentally, there is no evidence that babies who lie on their backs will choke if they happen to be sick, as used to be assumed.

Never let anyone smoke near a baby and, if your baby appears at all unwell, always seek medical advice immediately.

The Postnatal Check

You will have been given an appointment to return to the hospital for a postnatal check-up at around six to eight weeks after the birth. At this visit you should expect to:

• Be weighed
• Have your urine tested
• Have your blood pressure checked
• Have a blood sample taken
• Have your stitches checked to see if the wound has healed
• You may also have an internal examination to check that your womb has gone back to its normal size
• You will probably have a cervical smear
• You should be immunized against rubella if you were found not to be immune before your pregnancy
• You should have the opportunity to discuss any problems with the doctor
• If you had gestational diabetes during pregnancy then you will have a glucose tolerance test to make sure that blood glucose levels are back to normal and that you have not developed full-blown diabetes.

Going Back to Making Love

There are no rules that dictate when you should or should not resume sexual relations, although your genital area is bound to be rather sore at first. If you have had a Caesarean, your scar may well feel painful for quite a while. Some women find they simply lose their libido after the birth; they may feel flabby and unattractive, their breasts often feel tender and tiredness certainly doesn't help. There are many reasons why sex may not seem an appealing prospect in those early weeks, yet many couples do resume love-making after a short time and find it enjoyable. The key to success is taking it very slowly and, of course, extremely gently. Helping your partner understand how you feel both physically and mentally is most important. You must be able to communicate with your partner and he should be totally understanding. If you have had stitches then do not attempt penetration until you feel absolutely comfortable. Exploration and foreplay will help you to gauge how you feel. Once you are able to have full intercourse, use a lubricating jelly as certain glands which lubricate the vaginal area may not start to function again for a while after the birth. Do remember that you will need contraception as soon as you resume love-making – it is possible to conceive even if your periods have not started again and you are breastfeeding.

Things You Need to Do

There are some tasks that you will need to carry out within a certain time after the birth of your baby:

- Register the birth and obtain the birth certificate. This must be done within six weeks if you live in England, Wales or Northern Ireland or within three weeks if you live in Scotland.
- Find out if you qualify for certain state benefits and supplements. Obtain forms FB8 or CH11A from Social Security. This should be done as soon as possible.
- If you have not already applied for maternity payments from the Social fund, do so now or you may lose it (see Chapter 3).
- You must inform your employer as to whether or not you wish to go back to work. The latest time that you may return is 29 weeks from the beginning of the week of the birth; you should write to your employer at least three weeks before returning to protect your rights to the job.
- If you have not already been in touch, contact your

diabetes clinic and arrange an appointment for a check-up.

Postnatal Exercises

To get back into shape as soon as possible, do some (or all!) of the exercises below as soon as you can manage after delivery. It's a good idea to spend short periods exercising several times a day rather than attempting one long session. Don't forget pelvic floor exercises (see Chapter 8) to help tighten these muscles and reduce the risk of dribbling urine when you cough or laugh. You may not feel like taking time out for exercising but it's definitely worth it in the end. If you have had a Caesarean you should check with your midwife as to when it would be safe to start exercising.

- Lie flat on your back, your feet together and your legs straight. Keep your arms by your sides.
- Raise your head to look at your toes but without straining your shoulders.
- Relax and then repeat the sequence 6 times.

- Lie flat on your back with your feet together and your legs straight. Keep your arms by your sides.
- Draw your right leg up at the waist, then stretch it back down again.
- Return to the starting position and relax.
- Repeat the sequence using the left leg.
- Return to the starting position and relax.
- Repeat the sequence with each leg 3 times.

- Lie flat on your back, your feet together and your knees bent. Keep your arms by your sides.
- Tighten the muscles in your abdomen.

- Reach across your body with your right arm and place your right hand flat beside your left hip. This will be difficult – your upper body will want to come up off the floor – but try to stay flat on your back.
- Return to your starting position and relax.
- Repeat the sequence using the left arm and the left hand.
- Return to the starting position and relax.
- Repeat with each hand 3 times.

- Lie flat on your back with your feet together and your knees bent.
- Tighten the muscles in the lower abdomen and in the buttocks so that the small of your back is flat against the floor.
- Keeping these muscles tight, tighten the muscles of the back passage and the vagina (the pelvic floor muscles). Imagine you are trying to stop urine in mid-flow – these are the muscles you want to strengthen.
- Slowly, relax all the muscles.
- Repeat the sequence 3 times.

- Every now and then during the day, check that your posture is upright and correct. When standing, your weight should be placed slightly forward, over the front of your feet. Keep your knees straight.
- Raise your rib cage and pull in the muscles of your abdomen as far as you can.
- Raise your head towards the ceiling but keep your shoulders relaxed.
- This exercise can be practised at frequent intervals during the day, whenever you are standing still for a moment.

- Sit on a stool with your back straight against a wall.
- Keep your feet flat on the floor, directly under your knees.
- Bend forward and touch your toes. Then slowly uncurl from the base of your spine to your head and neck.
- Relax, still sitting up straight, and then repeat the

sequence 3 times.

- Stand up straight, your feet slightly apart and your weight evenly balanced between them. Keep your arms by your sides.
- Raise your left arm in a half-circle and, at the same time, stretch over to the right.
- Slide your right hand down the side of your right leg. Make sure that you keep your back straight and your bottom tucked in, so that you can feel a gentle pull on the muscles on the left side of your waist.
- Repeat, using the right arm.
- Repeat the sequence with each arm, 3 times.

As each day passes you will find that coping with diabetes and a new baby gets easier. Once you get to the end of your particular tunnel you will come out of the experience a new person. The challenge of coping with diabetes in pregnancy may have seemed like tackling the tallest mountain, but it is one that you will have climbed and, we very much hope, conquered. This is the time to congratulate yourself – for having the self-will to bring a healthy baby into the world. Now hopefully you will have the confidence to do it all over again.

We asked Debbie – who has had diabetes for 13 years and has two sons aged 7 and 5 – how she is coping with diabetes and family life now:

Great – the boys are both fine and healthy. Everything is second nature to me now – I might even consider another one!

USEFUL ADDRESSES

Below are some contacts covering many aspects of diabetes and pregnancy which you may find helpful.

British Diabetic Association (BDA)
10 Queen Anne Street
London W1M 0BD
071–323 1531
National organization providing links between people who have diabetes and their families, and publishing the latest information on care and treatment

National Childbirth Trust
Alexandra House
Oldham Terrace
London W0 6NII
081–992 8637

Pregnancy Advice

British Pregnancy Advisory Service (BPAS)
Austy Manor
Wootton
Warren
Solihull
West Midlands B95 6BX
05642 3225

Brook Advisory Centres
Central Office
233 Tottenham Court Road
London W1P 9AE
071–323 1522

**The Family Planning
Association**
27 Mortimer Street
London W1N 7RJ
071–636 7866

Health Education Authority
Hamilton House
Mabledon Place
London WC1H 9TX
071–383 3833

Postnatal Support

**Association of Breastfeeding
Mothers**
26 Holmshaw Close
London SE26 4TH
081–778 4769

**Birthright (National Fund
for Childbirth Research)**
27 Sussex Place
Regents Park
London NW1 4SP
071–723 9296

Caesarean Support Group
81 Elizabeth Way
Cambridge CB4 1BQ
0223 314811

The Maternity Alliance
15 Britannia Street
London WC1
071–837 1265

**The Meet-a-Mum
Association (MAMA)**
c/o 5 Westbury Gardens
Luton
Bedfordshire LU2 7DW
0582 422253

**Twins and Multiple Births
Association**
41 Fortuna Way
Aylesbury Park
Grimsby
South Humberside DN37 93J

Single Parents

Gingerbread
35 Wellington Street
London WC2 7BN
071–240 0953

**National Council for One
Parent Families**
255 Kentish Town Road
London NW5 2LX
071–267 1361

Bereavement Counselling

The Foundation for the Study of Infant Deaths
(Cot Death Research and Support)
5th Floor
4 Grosvenor Place
London SW1X 7HD
071–235 1721/245 9421

The Miscarriage Association
Dolphin Cottage
4 Ashfield Terrace
Thorpe
Wakefield
West Yorkshire
0532 828946

Stillbirth and Neonatal Death Society
37 Christchurch Hill
London NW3 1LA
071–794 4601

Blood Glucose Testing Equipment

Bayer Diagnostics UK
Ames Division
Evans House
Hamilton Close
Basingstoke
Hants RG21 2YE
0256 29181

Boehringer Mannheim UK
Bell Lane
Lewes
East Sussex BN7 1LG
0273 480444

Hypoguard (UK) Ltd
Dock Lane
Melton
Woodbridge
Suffolk IP12 1PE
03943 87333/4

Lifescan
Enterprise House
Station Road
Loudwater
High Wycombe
Bucks HP10 9UF
0494 450423

MediSense Britain Ltd
17 The Courtyard
Gorsey Lane
Coles Hill
Birmingham B46 1JA
0675 467044
Makes Exactech blood glucose testing equipment including pen sensor

Owen Mumford Ltd
(Medical Shop)
Brook Hill
Woodstock
Oxford OX7 1TU
0993 812021
Blood glucose testing equipment and accessories. Contact them for a brochure which includes all kinds of carrying equipment

Needles and Syringes

Becton Dickinson
Between Towns Road
Cowley
Oxford OX4 3LY
0865 777722

Insulin Manufacturers

Eli Lilly and Company Ltd
Kingsclere Road
Basingstoke
Hants RG21 2XA
0256 473241

**Novo Nordisk
Pharmaceuticals Ltd**
Novo Nordisk House
Broadfield Park
Brighton Road
Pease Pottage
Crawley
West Sussex RH11 9RT
0293 613555

Identification Jewellery

Medic-Alert Foundation
12 Bridge Wharf
156 Caledonian Road
London N1 9RD
071–833 3034

SOS/Talisman
Golden Key Co Ltd
1 Hare Street
Sheerness
Kent
ME12 1AH

Nappy Services

**National Association of
Nappy Services (NANS)**
Ground Floor
Kensington House
Suffolk Street
Queensway
Birmingham B1 1LN
021–693 4949
For details of the nappy laundering
service nearest you

BIBLIOGRAPHY

Nutritional Sub-committee of the Professional Advisory Committee, British Diabetic Association, 'Dietary Recommendations for People with Diabetes: An Update for the 1990s', *Diabetic Medicine* vol. 9, no. 2, 1992

Tina Healey and Mary Fodoor, *History of the Diabetic Diet* (Toronto: University of Toronto Press, 1992)

The authors are also grateful to the British Diabetic Association, the Department of Health and the Health Education Council for information and literature.

INDEX

187